RESPIRATORY CARE:
Know the Facts

RESPIRATORY CARE:
Know the Facts

Cynthia L. Howder, R.R.T., C.P.F.T.
St. Joseph's Hospital,
Tacoma, Washington
Illustrated by Steven E. Howder

J. B. Lippincott Company Philadelphia
London • New York • Mexico City • St. Louis
São Paulo • Sydney

Acquisitions Editor: *Charles McCormick, Jr.*
Manuscript Editor: *Lori J. Bainbridge*
Production Editor: *Linda J. Stewart*
Designer: *Anita Curry*
Production Manager: *Kathleen P. Dunn*
Production Assistant: *Pamela Milcos*
Compositor: *Bi–Comp*
Printer/Binder: *R. R. Donnelley*

6 5 4 3 2 1

Library of Congress Cataloging-in-Publication Data

Howder, Cynthia L.
  Respiratory care.

  Bibliography: p.
  1. Respiratory therapy—Handbooks, manuals, etc.
I. Title. [DNLM: 1. Respiratory Therapy.
2. Respiratory Tract Diseases—therapy.   WF 145 H854r]
RC735.I5H69 1989   616.2'0046   88-9264
ISBN 0-397-50940-5

Any procedure or practice described in this book should be applied
by the health-care practitioner under appropriate supervision in
accordance with professional standards of care used with regard to
the unique circumstances that apply in each practice situation. Care
has been taken to confirm the accuracy of information presented
and to describe generally accepted practices. However, the author,
editors, and publisher cannot accept any responsibility for errors or
omissions or for consequences from application of the information
in this book and make no warranty, express or implied, with re-
spect to the contents of the book.

Every effort has been made to ensure drug selections and dosages
are in accordance with current recommendations and practice.
Because of ongoing research, changes in government regulations
and the constant flow of information on drug therapy, reactions and
interactions, the reader is cautioned to check the package insert for
each drug for indications, dosages, warnings and precautions,
particularly if the drug is new or infrequently used.

This book is affectionately dedicated to

my husband Steve

and to my children,

Christina, Steven, Stephanie, Keven, and Kenny

preface

Respiratory care has come a long way since its recognition as a health care specialty. Practitioners are not only responsible to know all aspects of respiratory care, but all related therapy necessary for complete patient care as well. The material contained in *Respiratory Care: Know the Facts* was collected from numerous sources in an effort to present all the facts, figures, and equations necessary for total respiratory care.

In the course of daily clinical activities, the practitioner is required to recollect methods previously learned and facts not committed to memory. The major objective of *Respiratory Care: Know the Facts* is to present a comprehensive reference directory to the clinician. The concise outline style augments the usefulness of the book as a quick reference guide.

A comprehensive review section is included at the end of the book for students to assess their levels of retention and to evaluate their areas of weakness. It should be particularly helpful in preparing for the CRTT (Certified Respiratory Therapy Technician) and RRT (Registered Respiratory Therapist) examinations.

Cynthia L. Howder, R.R.T., C.P.F.T.

acknowledgments

I extend my thanks to all my sources.

I would also like to thank
my instructors at
Vincennes University, Vincennes, Indiana,
and especially
Dr. Richard Stein
for his support and encouragement
during my student days.

contents

D

E

F

G

H

I

L

M

N

O

P

R

S

T

U

V

W

X

Z

RESPIRATORY CARE:
Know the Facts

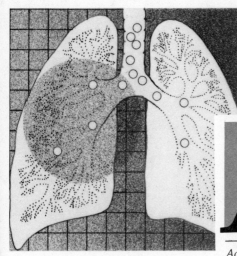

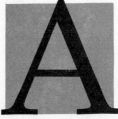

1

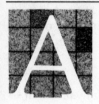

I. *Acid-Base Disorders*

A. Metabolic acidosis
  1. Uncompensated (acute)
     a. Decreased Hco_3^- (<22 mEq/L); decreased *p*H (<7.35)
  2. Compensated (chronic)
     a. Normal *p*H; decreased Hco_3^- with decreased $PaCO_2$
  3. Causes
     a. Diarrhea
        1) Depletion of bicarbonate through excretion
     b. Acetazolamide (Diamox)
        1) A carbonic anhydrase that prevents the reabsorption of Hco_3^- in the kidney
     c. Renal failure
        1) The kidney functions to excrete large quantities of acids without losing too much Hco_3^-

3

      2) In the presence of renal failure, the body's metabolic demands are not met, thereby creating the accumulation of blood acids and/or causing a decrease in the blood base level

  d. Lactic acidosis

      1) When oxygen is not readily available at the tissue level, anaerobic metabolism takes place, creating an increased formation of metabolic acids (lactic acidosis)

      2) Conditions that may cause anaerobic metabolism are circulatory insufficiency, reduced cardiac output, or severe hypoxemia (a result of an inadequate oxygen supply at the tissue level)

  e. Ketoacidosis

      1) Ketoacids are produced from an increased fat metabolism in such conditions as starvation and diabetes mellitus

4. May be treated with sodium bicarbonate therapy

B. Metabolic alkalosis

1. Uncompensated (acute)

  a. Increased Hco_3^- (>26 mEq/L); increased pH (>7.45)

2. Compensated (chronic)

  a. Normal pH; increased Hco_3^- with increased $PaCO_2$

3. Causes

  a. Loss of acids (loss of hydrogen ion)

      1) Conditions that create a depletion of hydrogen ion are nasogastric suctioning and vomiting

    b. Hypokalemia

       1) Decreased intracellular K^+ causes H^+ to diffuse intracellularly (to maintain an electric balance)

       2) The result is insufficient free H^+ levels extracellularly, creating an alkalosis

    c. Diuretics

       1) Promote the excretion of K^+, resulting in hypokalemia

    d. Hypochloremia

       1) Decreased extracellular chloride levels cause intracellular Hco_3^- to shift extracellularly, creating an excess of blood Hco_3^-

4. May be treated with acetazolamide to promote bicarbonate excretion in the urine

C. Respiratory acidosis

  1. Uncompensated (acute)

    a. Increased $PaCO_2$ (>50 mm Hg); decreased pH (<7.35)

  2. Compensated (chronic)

    a. Normal pH; increased $PaCO_2$ with increased Hco_3^-

  3. Causes

    a. Respiratory failure

       1) Respiratory center depression

       2) Decreased oxygen consumption efficiency

       3) Decreased ventilatory reserve

       4) Ventilatory muscle fatigue or failure

    b. End stage cardiopulmonary disease

       1) Severe gas exchange abnormality

       2) Chronic CO_2 retention

       3) Compromised cardiopulmonary status

c. Central nervous system (CNS) depression
   1) Abnormal ventilatory center depression by drugs, trauma, or tumor
   2) Results in alveolar hypoventilation, and acidosis
4. Treatment aimed at correcting underlying cause; possible mechanical ventilation

D. Respiratory alkalosis
1. Uncompensated (acute)
   a. Decreased $PaCO_2$ (<35 mm Hg); increased pH (>7.45)
2. Compensated (chronic)
   a. Normal pH; decreased $PaCO_2$ with decreased HCO_3^-
3. Causes
   a. CNS stimulation
      1) Increased stimulation of the ventilatory centers by drugs, trauma, or tumor
      2) Results in alveolar hyperventilation, alkalosis
   b. Pain, anxiety, fear, hysteria
      1) Emotional disorders generate hyperventilation
   c. Hypoxemia
      1) The compensatory mechanism for hypoxemia is hyperventilation by stimulation of the peripheral chemoreceptors
4. Treatment aimed at correcting underlying cause

II. Aerosol Therapy

A. Suspended liquid or solid particles
B. Goals

    1. Promote bronchial hygiene

    2. Liquify secretions

    3. Humidify dry gases

    4. Deliver medication

C. Hazards

    1. Bronchospasm

    2. Swelling of secretions

    3. Fluid overload

    4. Cross contamination

D. Aerosol solutions

    1. Hypertonic

       a. Particle size increases in airway

       b. Indicated for sputum induction

    2. Isotonic

       a. Particle size remains stable

       b. Indicated for small volume nebulizers

    3. Hypotonic

       a. Particle size decreases in airway

       b. Least effect on airway resistance

E. Volume output, factors affecting

    1. Size of particles

    2. Number of particles

    3. Flow

       a. High flow

          1) Increased air entrainment

          2) Greater output

          3) Decreased density

       b. Low flow

          1) Decreased air entrainment

          2) Decreased output

          3) Increased density

    c. Total flow
       1) Need minimum three times patient's minute volume
       2) Inadequate total flow will cause increased air entrainment by the patient entraining ambient room air to meet the total inspiratory demand

F. *Particle size (μ)*   *Deposition site*

1. 100 to 5   Trapped in nose; larynx
2. 5 to 2   Bronchioles
3. 2 to 1   To alveoli
4. 1 to 0.25   Enters alveoli
5. 0.25   Alveolar deposition
6. 0.1   Inhaled and exhaled

G. Infection control
   1. Heated aerosol
     a. Increased risk for nosocomial infection
       1) Bacteria grow well in humidified environments
     b. Aerosol unit to be changed daily

III. Airway Management

A. Indications
   1. Provide a patent airway
   2. Guard the airway from aspiration
   3. Provide ease of suctioning
   4. Promote mechanical ventilation

B. Airway cuffs
   1. Indications

   a. Promote mechanical ventilation
   b. Guard the airway from aspiration
2. Cuff pressure effects
   a. 5 mm Hg: lymph system impairment
   b. 18 mm Hg: venous system impairment
   c. 25 mm Hg: arterial system impairment
3. Types of cuffs
   a. Low residual volume; high pressure
      1) Produces wall pressures of 40 to 200 mm Hg
      2) Use the minimal leak technique to reduce the possibility of capillary blood occlusion
   b. High residual volume; low pressure
      1) Produces wall pressures of 25 mm Hg or less
      2) Reduces necrotic effect
   c. Fome cuff
      1) Produces wall pressures of 20 mm Hg or less
      2) Self-inflating
4. Hazards
   a. Impaired tracheal blood flow (ischemia)
   b. Tracheal softening; collapse (malacia)
   c. Tracheal constriction (stenosis)
C. Oral pharyngeal airway
   1. Complications
      a. If too long
         1) Occludes larynx
         2) Causes gastric insufflation
      b. If too short
         1) Airway occlusion by tongue
   2. Used mainly for comatose patients

D. Nasal pharyngeal airway
   1. Terminal portion positioned at the base of the tongue
   2. Preferred airway for semicomatose or aware patients

IV. Alveoloarterial Gradient ($A - aDO_2$)

A. Gives a rough estimate of the percent shunt
B. Normal value 10 to 20 mm Hg
C. Equation: $P_AO_2 - PaO_2$
D. Normal value found with hypoxemia and
   1. Hypoventilation
   2. Increased altitude
E. Increased value found with hypoxemia and
   1. Shunt
   2. V/Q mismatch
   3. Diffusion defect
F. For every 20 mm Hg gradient; approximately a 1% shunt exists

V. Arterial Blood Gas Sampling

A. Sites in order of preference
   1. Radial (perform Allen test for collateral circulation; tests the patency of the ulnar artery)
   2. Brachial
   3. Femoral

B. Sample with air bubble

1. $Paco_2$ decreases (high blood Pco_2 diffuses out into the low air Pco_2); pH will correspondingly increase

2. PaO_2 may increase or decrease

   a. $PaO_2 > 159$ mm Hg; PaO_2 decreases (high blood Po_2 diffuses out to equalize air/blood Po_2)

   b. $PaO_2 < 159$ mm Hg; PaO_2 increases (air Po_2 diffuses into blood sample to equalize gradient)

C. Temperature correction

1. Hyperthermic patient (right shifted HbO_2 curve)

   a. PaO_2 and $PaCO_2$ will be lower than actual value if measured in a 37°C blood gas machine

   b. pH will be greater than actual value

2. Hypothermic patient (left shifted HbO_2 curve)

   a. PaO_2 and $PaCO_2$ will be higher than actual value if measured in a 37°C blood gas machine

   b. pH will be less than actual value

D. Sample not iced

1. Metabolic activity remains

   a. Causes an increased $PaCO_2$

   b. Causes a decreased pH, PaO_2

E. Heparin

1. Sodium heparin commonly used in blood gas syringes

   a. 0.05 ml sodium heparin to 1 ml blood

   b. Increased volume of heparin in syringe, or a small blood volume

      1) $PaCO_2$ value will decrease

      2) pH value decreases

      3) PaO_2 may increase or decrease depending on heparin's Po_2 level and blood Po_2 level

  2. Ammonium heparin is not used because its pH will affect blood's pH level

VI. Arteriovenous Gradient ($a - vDO_2$)

A. Assesses tissue oxygenation

B. Normal value 5 vol%

C. Equation: $CaO_2 - CvO_2$

  1. $a - vDO_2 = (1.34 \times Hb \times HBO_2 \text{ arterial}) + (0.003 \times PaO_2) - (1.34 \times Hb \times HbO_2 \text{ venous}) + (0.003 \times PvO_2)$

D. Increased value found with circulatory hypoxia

  1. Slow blood transit time results in greater depletion of the oxygen content, creating a wider difference in the $a - vDO_2$

E. Decreased value found with histotoxic hypoxia

  1. Oxygen not released at the tissue level causes both the arterial and the venous oxygen contents to remain nearly the same

VII. Assessment of Patient

A. Collect patient data

B. Interview and observe patient

C. Assess perfusion

1. Urine output
    a. <30 ml/hr; decreased perfusion
2. Skin
    a. Warm and dry; adequate perfusion
    b. Cold and clammy; decreased perfusion
3. Capillary refill time
4. Sensorium
5. Peripheral pulses

D. Examine chest
1. Inspection
    a. Breathing pattern
    b. Chest wall structure
2. Palpation (see Palpation Technique)
3. Percussion (see Percussion Notes)
4. Auscultation (see Breath Sounds)

VIII. Atmospheric Pressure Conversion and Composition

A. One atmosphere is equal to
1. 760 mm Hg
2. 76 cm Hg
3. 1034 g/cm^2
4. 1034 cm H_2O
5. 14.7 psi
6. 29 in Hg
7. 33 ft H_2O

B. Composition of the atmosphere

1. | Gas | % |
   |---|---|
   | a. Nitrogen | 79 |
   | b. Oxygen | 21 |
   | c. Argon | 0.93 |
   | d. Carbon dioxide | 0.03 |

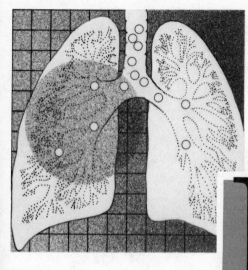

B

Blood Pressure

Blood Values

Breath Sounds

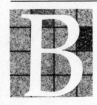

I. Blood Pressure

A. Systolic—left ventricular status
1. Highest pressure reading taken from the artery
2. Normal values (mm Hg)
    a. Neonate   80
    b. 1 to 2 year old   90
    c. Child   90 to 110
    d. Teenager   90 to 125
    e. Adult   90 to 140

B. Diastolic—peripheral resistance
1. Lowest pressure reading taken from the artery
2. Normal values (mm Hg)
    a. Neonate   46
    b. 1 to 2 year old   60
    c. Child   60 to 72
    d. Teenager   60 to 80
    e. Adult   60 to 90

C. Pulse pressure
1. Difference existing between systolic and diastolic pressures

    2. Normally an increased value indicates an increase in blood flow
- **D.** Treatment for hypertension
  1. Propranolol HCL (Inderal)
  2. Nitroprusside (Nipride)
  3. Diazoxide (Hyperstat)
- **E.** Treatment for hypotension
  1. Dopamine
  2. Placing patient in Trendelenburg position

II. *Blood Values*

- **A.** Arterial blood gas values for normal patients
  1. $PaCO_2$ — 35 to 45 mm Hg
  2. PaO_2 — 80 to 100 mm Hg
  3. pH — 7.35 to 7.45
  4. Hco_3^- — 22 to 26 mEq/L
  5. Base excess — -2 to $+2$
  6. Hemoglobin — 14 to 16 mg/dl
  7. Saturation — 97%
  8. O_2 content — 20 vol%
- **B.** Venous blood gas values for normal patients
  1. $PvCO_2$ — 46 mm Hg
  2. PvO_2 — 40 mm Hg
  3. pH — 7.35
  4. Saturation — 75%
  5. O_2 content — 16 vol%
- **C.** Blood volume
  1. 70 ml/kg
  2. 5% to 7% of total body weight

D. Electrolytes
  1. Sodium   135–145 mEq/L
  2. Chloride   100–110 mEq/L
  3. Bicarbonate   24 to 30 mEq/L
  4. Potassium   3.5 to 5 mEq/L
  5. Calcium   4.5 to 5 mEq/L

E. Complete blood count (CBC)
  1. Red blood cells
      a. Female   4 to 5 million/μl
      b. Male   5 to 6 million/μl
  2. White blood cells
      a. Male and female   5–10 thousand/μl
  3. Hematocrit
      a. Female   37 to 47 vol%
      b. Male   40 to 54 vol%
  4. Hemoglobin
      a. Normally one-third of hematocrit
      b. 14 to 16 g/100 ml

F. Miscellaneous blood values
  1. Sweat test
      a. Chloride   4 to 60 mEq/L
      b. Sodium   10 to 80 mEq/L
  2. Glucose   65 to 110 mg/100 ml
  3. Albumin   4 to 5.5 g/100 ml
  4. Platelets   200,000–350,000/mm^3

III. Breath Sounds

A. Tracheal breath sounds
  1. Heard over the trachea
  2. Harsh, tubular sound

B. Bronchial breath sounds
  1. Heard only over the manubrium
  2. Tubular, hollow sound
  3. Abnormal bronchial breath sounds (heard in areas of the chest other than stated above) are present when alveoli are fluid filled, collapsed, or replaced with solid tissue
     a. Atelectasis
     b. Pneumonia
     c. Pulmonary infarction

C. Vesicular breath sounds
  1. Heard over most areas of the chest except directly over the trachea and bronchi
  2. Breezy sound

D. Bronchovesicular breath sounds
  1. Normally heard over the upper sternum, both sides of the sternum, and between the scapulae
  2. Breezy, muffled sound
  3. Abnormal bronchovesicular breath sounds (heard in areas of the chest other than stated above) are present when there is a reduction (but not a total loss) in ventilating tissue
     a. Early pneumonia
     b. Pulmonary edema

E. Absent breath sounds
  1. No air transmission through loss of ventilating lung or by total obstruction
     a. Pleural effusion
     b. Pneumothorax
     c. Atelectasis
     d. Paralyzed diaphragm
     e. Foreign body

F. Adventitious breath sounds

    1. Rales

        a. Musical

            1) Continuous dry rales

            2) Types

                a) Sibilant—wheeze; occurs in small airways

                b) Sonorous—snoring; occurs in larger airways

        b. Crepitant

            1) Moist rales

            2) Heard during inspiration

    2. Rhonchi

        a. Coarse, rattling sound

        b. Usually heard during expiration

        c. Sometimes clears after a cough

    3. Gurgling rales/rhonchi

        a. Copious amounts of secretions lodged in the upper airway

        b. Known as the "death rattle"

G. Nonpulmonic sounds

    1. Pleural friction rub

        a. Grating sound heard when the pleural surfaces rub together

        b. Conditions that cause the pleura to become inflamed

            1) Acute infections

            2) Pleural effusion

            3) Pulmonary infarction

    2. Subcutaneous emphysema

        a. Air trapped under the skin; produces a popping sound when palpated

  b. Not synonymous with the respiratory cycle
  c. Conditions that may trap free air in or
     around the subcutaneous tissues
     1) Pneumothorax
     2) Lung punctures
     3) Neck surgery
     4) Tracheostomy

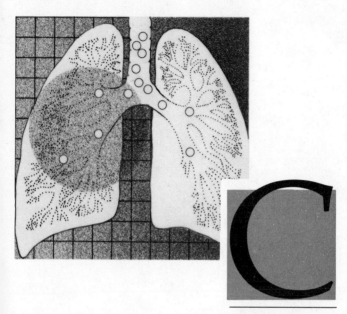

C

Chemoreceptors

Chest Tubes

Concentrators

Constant Positive
Airway Pressure
(CPAP) Therapy

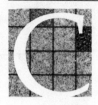

I. Chemoreceptors

A. Peripheral
  1. Located in carotid, aortic bodies
  2. Responds to decreased levels of PaO_2 (<60 mm Hg)
  3. Activation causes an increase in ventilation
  4. Does not adapt to chronic levels of hypoxemia
B. Central
  1. Located in the medulla
  2. Responds to an increased level of $PaCO_2$, or a change in the pH of the cerebral spinal fluid
  3. Activation causes an increase in ventilation
  4. Adapts to chronic hypercapnia
     a. Inactivates the need for increased ventilation
C. Hypoxic drive
  1. Primarily found in chronic hypercapnic and hypoxemic patients
  2. Increasing the level of PaO_2 with supplemental oxygen diminishes the need for stimulated ventilation

   3. Result is somnolence, lethargy, and further
      increasing $PaCO_2$

II. Chest Tubes

A. Directs air/fluid from the pleura
   1. Re-expands the lung by establishing subatmos-
      pheric pressure in the pleura
   2. One-way valve system that prevents atmo-
      spheric pressure from gaining entry into the
      pleura
B. Suction maintained by the amount of water in the
   suction control chamber
C. Precautions
   1. Clamping of chest tube may cause tension
      pneumothorax
   2. If bubbling ceases
      a. No longer an air leak present
      b. Obstructed tubing
   3. Excessive bubbling
      a. Large pneumothorax present
      b. Leak in system
   4. Always set drainage system below the level of
      the chest
   5. If underwater seal bottle breaks
      a. Immerse chest tube in a container of water
      b. Never attach directly to a suction system
D. Simple underwater seal
   1. Not attached to suction source
   2. Can transport or ambulate patient

E. Placement for a pneumothorax
   1. Third or fourth intercostal space
   2. Midaxillary line
   3. Directed toward apex
F. Placement for a hemothorax
   1. Sixth or seventh intercostal space
   2. Midaxillary or postaxillary line
   3. Directed posteriorly

III. *Concentrators*

A. Permeable plastic membrane
   1. Oxygen and P_{H_2O} pass through faster than nitrogen
   2. Result is humidified 40% oxygen at 1 to 10 LPM
   3. Actual liter flow needs to be increased to compensate for receiving only 40% oxygen
B. Molecular sieve
   1. Silicate absorbs nitrogen
   2. Oxygen concentration depends on flowrate
      a. 2 LPM; 90% oxygen
      b. 10 LPM; 50% oxygen

IV. *Constant Positive Airway Pressure (CPAP) Therapy*

A. Indications
   1. Refractory hypoxemia
      a. $PaO_2 < 50$ mm Hg; $FiO_2 > 0.6$

    2. Pulmonary edema

    3. Hyaline membrane disease (HMD)

    4. Adult respiratory distress syndrome (ARDS)

    5. Chest trauma

    6. Atelectasis

B. Goals

    1. Increase functional residual capacity (FRC)

    2. Improve oxygenation

    3. Maintain a $PaO_2 > 50$ mm Hg with an $FIO_2 < 0.5$

C. Hazards

    1. Gastric distention

    2. Vomiting

    3. Aspiration

    4. Patient discomfort

D. Monitoring

    1. Hourly measurements of blood pressure and pulse

    2. Arterial blood gas (ABG) analysis within 1 hr after the initiation of CPAP

    3. Monitor cardiac output for a decreased value

    4. Analyze FIO_2 with an oxygen analyzer

    5. Analyze CPAP setting with a pressure or water manometer

E. Devices

    1. Mask (must be a tight fit)

    2. Nasal prongs

       a. Used for neonates

       b. Obligatory nose breathers

    3. Endotracheal tube

F. Maintaining nonfluctuating CPAP
  1. Flow
     a. Minimum three times patient's minute volume
     b. Measured distal to the CPAP device

G. CPAP/PEEP (positive end expiratory pressure) valves
  1. Simple water column
     a. Amount of water in container equals PEEP generated

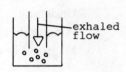

  2. Spring loaded
     a. Ambu
     b. Servo B (external attachment)

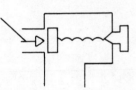

  3. Pressurized exhalation diaphragm
     a. Bear I
     b. Bear II
     c. Gill-1

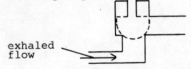

  4. Venturi opposing flow
     a. Bear Cub
     b. BP-200

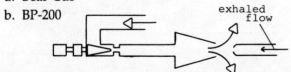

5. Spring and diaphragm with pressurized balloon
   a. Ma-1

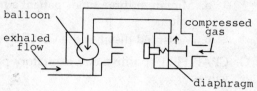

6. Underwater seal
7. Weighted ball
8. Magnetic force

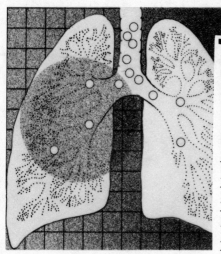

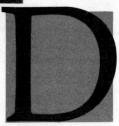

31

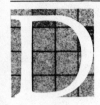

I. *Deadspace* (V_D)

A. Ventilation exceeding perfusion
B. Normal value 20% to 40%
C. Calculated by the Bohr equation

   1. $V_D/V_t = \dfrac{PaCO_2 - P_ECO_2}{PaCO_2}$

D. Anatomic V_D
   1. Ventilation that is not in contact with alveoli
   2. 1 ml/pound
   3. Normally 150 ml
E. Alveolar V_D
   1. Ventilation that is in contact with nonperfused alveoli
F. Physiologic V_D
   1. Sum of anatomic V_D plus alveolar V_D
G. Conditions that cause an increase in V_D
   1. Mechanical ventilation (increased ventilation)
   2. Myocardial infarction (impaired cardiac perfusion)

3. Hemorrhage (decreased perfusion)
4. Pulmonary emboli (low alveolar capillary perfusion)

II. Diseases: Neonatal

A. IRDS
   1. Synonymous names
      a. Idiopathic respiratory distress syndrome
      b. Hyaline membrane disease
   2. Etiology
      a. Decreased L/S ratio
      b. Decreased surfactant production
      c. Associated with premature birth
   3. Clinical findings
      a. Grunting
      b. Nasal flaring
      c. Intercostal retractions
      d. Rapid respiratory rates
   4. Chest x-ray
      a. Ground glass presentation
      b. Air bronchogram
   5. Pathophysiology
      a. Atelectasis
      b. Decreased compliance; decreased functional residual capacity (FRC)
      c. Right to left shunting
      d. Severe hypoxemia
   6. Treatment
      a. Maintaining PaO_2 between 50 to 70 mm Hg

        1) Least FiO_2 necessary

        2) CPAP therapy

    b. Ventilatory management when necessary

    c. Maintain adequate cardiovascular stability

    d. Reduce the amount of stress to the neonate

B. Bronchopulmonary dysplasia (BPD)

    1. Disease that accompanies ventilatory therapy

      a. High FiO_2

      b. High mean airway pressures

    2. Pathophysiology

      a. Chronic pulmonary changes

      b. Interstitial fibrosis

C. Transient tachypnea of the newborn

    1. Continual high respiratory rates

    2. Diagnosis

      a. Chest x-ray

        1) Central perihilar markings

        2) Slightly enlarged cardiac silhouette

    3. Pathophysiology

      a. Slow absorption of fetal lung fluid

      b. Decreased lung compliance

    4. Self-limiting disease

      a. Usually resolves in 3 to 4 days

III. Diseases: Neuromuscular

A. Myasthenia gravis

    1. Neuromuscular dysfunction in which there is inhibition of impulse transmission

    2. Generalized muscle weakness—descending pattern

   3. Etiology
      a. Thought to be improperly released acetyl-choline
   4. Treatment
      a. Parasympathomimetics
      b. Atropine
      c. Monitoring forced vital capacity (FVC)
B. Guillain–Barré
   1. Neuron inflammation resulting in abnormal peripheral motor and sensory neuron function
   2. Ascending pattern of paralysis
   3. Etiology
      a. Unknown, cases reported following influenza vaccinations or viral illness
   4. Diagnosis
      a. Increased protein content in the cerebral spinal fluid
   5. Treatment
      a. Supportive with possible ventilatory management
      b. Disease is reversible

IV. Diseases: Obstructive

A. Asthma
   1. Reversible disease that causes an increased irritability of the trachea and bronchi to various stimuli
   2. Laboratory findings
      a. Curschmann's spirals

   b. Eosinophils
   c. Charcot–Leyden crystals
3. ABG stages

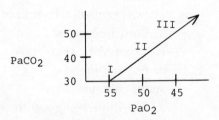

As the hypoxemia becomes severe (from pronounced obstruction), a critical point is reached where the patient begins to show fatigue; resulting in increasing $PaCO_2$s—ventilatory failure
   a. Phase I—initial distress
      1) PaO_2 and $PaCO_2$ decreased; pH increased
   b. Phase II—impending respiratory failure
      1) PaO_2 decreased; $PaCO_2$ and pH normal
   c. Phase III—respiratory failure
      1) PaO_2 and pH decreased; $PaCO_2$ increased
4. Physical findings
   a. Prolonged expiration with wheezes
   b. Rapid respiratory rates with hypoventilation
   c. Use of accessory muscles
   d. Increased dyspnea with decreased wheezing
      1) Silent chest; impending respiratory failure
   e. Tachycardia
   f. Hypertension
5. Response to therapy guided by FEV_1, peak flow

6. Disease shows a normal $D_{L_{CO}}$
7. Chest x-ray
   a. Hyperinflation
8. Treatment
   a. Environmental control of irritating stimuli
   b. Bronchodilators
   c. Theophylline
   d. Oxygen therapy
9. Status asthmaticus
   a. Life-threatening asthmatic attack that does not respond to conventional therapy
   b. Treatment
      1) Intravenous corticosteroids
      2) Mechanical ventilation when indicated

B. Bronchiectasis
   1. Nonreversible disease characterized by distorted and distended bronchi
   2. Classification
      a. Cylindrical
         1) Usually follows severe chronic bronchitis
         2) Abnormal distended bronchial walls
      b. Fusiform
         1) Associated with many large irregular bronchial dilations
      c. Saccular
         1) Advanced form with worst prognosis
         2) Total deterioration of bronchial walls
   3. Laboratory findings
      a. Three-layer sputum

4. Physical findings
    a. Chronic productive cough
    b. Repeated pulmonary infections
    c. Malnutrition
    d. Digital clubbing
5. Chest x-ray
    a. Scattered small cavities
    b. Air bronchogram
6. Treatment
    a. Vigorous bronchial hygiene
    b. Postural drainage
    c. Antibiotics for infection

C. Bronchitis
    1. Acute
        a. Excessive mucus production with irritation and inflammation of the bronchi
    2. Chronic
        a. Excessive mucus production accompanied with a chronic cough for 3 months per year for 2 or more years
    3. Physical findings
        a. Continual cough
        b. Mucopurulent sputum
        c. Irritated, inflamed, and edematous airways
    4. Chest x-ray
        a. Hyperinflation
        b. Flattening of the diaphragm
    5. Treatment
        a. Environmental control

    b. Bronchodilator therapy
    c. Postural drainage
    d. Antibiotics

D. Emphysema
  1. Disease characterized by abnormal, distended alveoli with loss of lung elastance
  2. Classification
    a. Centrilobular
      1) Involves upper lobes
      2) Smoking
      3) Bronchitis
    b. Panlobular
      1) Involves lower lobes
      2) Natural aging
      3) Alpha$_1$ antitrypsin deficiency
  3. Physical findings
    a. Recurrent respiratory infections
    b. Digital clubbing
    c. Barrel chest
    d. Use of accessory muscles
    e. Irritating nonproductive cough
  4. Chest x-ray
    a. Hyperinflation
    b. Flattened diaphragm
  5. Treatment
    a. Bronchodilators
    b. Postural drainage
    c. Antibiotics
    d. Supplemental oxygen for hypoxemia
    e. Education and support

V. *Diseases: Pediatric*

A. Epiglottitis
1. Acute upper airway obstruction
2. Life-threatening disease
3. Diagnosis
   a. Lateral x-ray of neck
      1) Epiglottis swollen
      2) Subglottic area normal
4. Etiology
   a. *Hemophilus influenzae*
5. Physical findings
   a. Inspiratory stridor
   b. Fever
   c. Dyspnea
   d. Intercostal retractions
6. Treatment
   a. Intubation
   b. Antibiotics for *H. influenzae*
      1) Chloramphenicol
      2) Ampicillin
B. Laryngotracheobronchitis—viral croup
1. Inflammation and irritation to the upper airway
2. Diagnosis
   a. Lateral x-ray of neck
      1) Epiglottis normal
      2) Subglottic narrowing
3. Etiology
   a. Parainfluenza virus
   b. Adenovirus
   c. Respiratory syncytial virus

4. Physical findings
   a. Inspiratory stridor
   b. Dry, croupy cough
   c. Fever
5. Treatment
   a. Cool mist therapy
   b. Racemic epinephrine

C. Cystic fibrosis—mucoviscidosis
1. Disease characterized by dysfunctioning exocrine gland
2. Etiology
   a. Inherited autosomal recessive gene
3. Diagnosis
   a. Positive sweat test (>60 mEq/L)
4. Clinical findings
   a. Bulky, foul-smelling stools
   b. Protruding abdomen
   c. Barrel chested
   d. Digital clubbing
5. Repeated infections are most life-threatening
6. Treatment
   a. Vigorous bronchial hygiene
      1) Aerosol therapy
      2) Postural drainage
      3) Mucolytics
   b. Antibiotics when infection is present

VI. Diseases: Restrictive

A. ARDS
1. Restrictive disease that follows damage to the lungs (directly or indirectly)

2. Synonymous names
   a. Adult respiratory distress syndrome
   b. Congestive atelectasis
   c. Shock lung
   d. Stiff lung syndrome
   e. Capillary leak syndrome
3. Latent period of 12 to 24 hours from the occurrence of lung injury to the manifestation of ARDS
4. Physical findings
   a. Respiratory distress
   b. Severe hypoxemia
   c. High minute volumes, rapid respiratory rates
5. Pathophysiology
   a. Refractory hypoxemia
   b. Decreased FRC
   c. Decreased lung compliance
   d. Atelectasis
   e. Noncardiogenic pulmonary edema
6. Chest x-ray
   a. Diffuse bilateral infiltrates
   b. Honeycomb appearance
7. Treatment
   a. Mechanical ventilation with PEEP
   b. Proper fluid management
   c. Methylprednisolone sodium succinate (Solu-Medrol)

B. Pulmonary Edema—Noncardiogenic
   1. Disease following the transference of fluid from the interstitial space to the alveoli, resulting in pulmonary congestion

   2. Conditions that may result in pulmonary edema owing to an abnormal alveolar capillary membrane permeability
      a. Drug overdose
      b. Smoke inhalation
      c. Toxic gas inhalation
      d. Aspiration
      e. Near drowning
   3. Pathophysiology
      a. Normal or decreased pulmonary capillary wedge pressure
      b. Increased capillary permeability
      c. Hypoxemia
   4. Chest x-ray
      a. Fluffy (butterfly) alveolar infiltrates
   5. Treatment
      a. PEEP therapy
C. Pulmonary edema—Cardiogenic
   1. Etiology
      a. Left ventricular failure
         1) The inability of the left heart to function normally creates an increased hydrostatic pressure in the pulmonary system, resulting in pulmonary congestion
   2. Pathophysiology
      a. Increased pulmonary capillary wedge pressure
      b. Increased hydrostatic pressure
   3. Chest x-ray
      a. Fluffy alveolar infiltrates
      b. Enlarged cardiac shadow

4. Treatment
    a. Furosemide (Lasix)
    b. Morphine sulfate
    c. Digitalis
    d. PEEP therapy

VII. Drugs: For Cardiac Arrest and Arrhythmia

A. Epinephrine
  1. Action
      a. Sympathomimetic drug secreted by the adrenal gland
      b. Positive inotropic effect
      c. Increases heart rate, systemic vascular resistance
      d. Stimulates spontaneous myocardial contractions
  2. Indications
      a. Anaphylactic shock
      b. Cardiac arrest
      c. Allergic reactions—bronchial asthma
  3. Side effects—overdose
      a. Ventricular fibrillation
      b. Hypertension
      c. Pulmonary edema
      d. Tachycardia
B. Atropine
  1. Action
      a. Parasympatholytic
      b. Improves atrial/ventricular conduction

    2. Indications

      a. Sinus bradycardia

      b. Ventricular asystole

    3. Side effects—overdose

      a. Dilated pupils

      b. Delirium

      c. Coma

      d. Tachycardia

C. Calcium chloride

    1. Action

      a. Increases ventricular regularity

      b. Positive inotropic effect

    2. Indications

      a. Hypocalcemia

      b. Cardiac resuscitation

    3. Side effects—overdose

      a. Arrhythmia

      b. Cardiac arrest

      c. Bradycardia

D. Lidocaine (Xylocaine)

    1. Action

      a. Decreases myocardial conduction

      b. Increases fibrillation threshold

    2. Indications

      a. PVC (premature ventricular contraction)

      b. V-tach (ventricular tachycardia)

      c. V-fib (ventricular fibrillation)

    3. Side effects—overdose

      a. Hypotension

      b. Respiratory arrest

      c. Cardiovascular collapse

E. Procainamide HCL (Pronestyl)
1. Action
   a. Same as Lidocaine
2. Indications
   a. Suppress PVC
   b. Uncontrollable V-tach
3. Side effects
   a. Hypotension
   b. Heart block; cardiac arrest
F. Sodium bicarbonate
1. Action
   a. Management of metabolic acidosis
2. Indication
   a. Metabolic acidosis
3. Side effects
   a. Metabolic alkalosis
   b. Post arrest cerebral impairment

VIII. Drugs: Cardiovascular

A. Dopamine (Intropin)
1. Action
   a. Positive inotropic effect
      1) Increases cardiac output
      2) Increases urine output
2. Indications
   a. Cardiogenic shock
   b. Hemodynamic hypotension
B. Dobutamine HCL (Dobutrex)
1. Action
   a. Short-term inotropic effect

2. Indication
    a. Used with Nipride to increase cardiac output and to decrease pulmonary capillary wedge pressure
C. Sodium Nitroprusside (Nipride)
    1. Action
        a. Antihypertensive agent
    2. Indication
        a. Reduction of blood pressure
D. Propranolol HCL (Inderal)
    1. Action
        a. Prolongs atrial/ventricular conduction
    2. Indications
        a. Supraventricular and atrial arrhythmias

IX. Drugs: Diuretics

A. Furosemide (Lasix)
    1. Action
        a. Diuretic—slows reabsorption of sodium
    2. Indications
        a. Pulmonary edema
        b. Edema
B. Mannitol
    1. Action
        a. Osmotic diuretic—slows reabsorption of water and solutes
    2. Indications
        a. Reduces intracranial pressure
        b. Enhances diuresis in acute renal failure

X. *Drugs: Narcotic Antagonist*

A. Naloxone HCL (Narcan)
  1. Action
     a. Narcotic antagonist
  2. Indications
     a. Reversal of narcotic depression
     b. Reversal of respiratory depression induced by narcotics

XI. *Drugs: Neuromuscular*

A. Pancuronium bromide (Pavulon) and Succinylcholine
  1. Action
     a. Neuromuscular blocking agent
  2. Indications
     a. To facilitate mechanical ventilatory management
     b. An aid to intubation

XII. *Drugs: Respiratory*

A. Sympathomimetics
  1. Epinephrine HCl
     a. Action
        1) Catecholamine
        2) Equal alpha and beta stimulation

    b. Strength
      1) 1 : 100; 10 mg/ml
    c. Dosage
      1) 0.25 to 0.5 ml in 3 ml saline
    d. Hazards
      1) Tachycardia
      2) Hypertension

2. Racemic epinephrine
    a. Action
      1) Catecholamine
      2) Equal alpha and beta stimulation
    b. Strength
      1) 2.25%; 22.5 mg/ml
    c. Dosage
      1) 0.25 to 0.5 ml in 3 ml saline
    d. Hazards
      1) Tachycardia
      2) Hypertension

3. Isoetharine (Bronkosol)
    a. Action
      1) Catecholamine
      2) Beta$_2$ stimulant
    b. Strength
      1) 1%; 10 mg/ml
    c. Dosage
      1) 0.25 to 0.5 ml in 3 ml saline
    d. Hazards
      1) Tachycardia
      2) Hypertension

XII. Drugs: Respiratory **51**

4. Isoproterenol HCL (Isuprel)
   a. Action
      1) Catecholamine
      2) Powerful $beta_1$ and $beta_2$ stimulant
   b. Strength
      1) 1:200; 5 mg/ml
   c. Dosage
      1) 0.25 to 0.5 ml in 3 ml saline
   d. Hazards
      1) Tachycardia
      2) Hypertension
5. Metaproterenol sulfate (Alupent, Metaprel)
   a. Action
      1) Resorcinol
      2) $Beta_2$ stimulant
   b. Strength
      1) 5%
   c. Dosage
      1) 0.2 to 0.3 ml in 3 ml saline
   d. Hazards
      1) Minimal cardiac stimulation
6. Terbutaline sulfate (Brethine, Bricanyl)
   a. Action
      1) Resorcinol
      2) $Beta_2$ stimulant
      3) Twice as potent as Alupent
   b. Strength
      1) 0.1%, 1 mg/ml
   c. Dosage
      1) 1 to 2 ml in 3 ml saline

      d. Hazards
        1) Minimal cardiac stimulation
   7. Albuterol sulfate (Ventolin, Proventil)
      a. Action
        1) Saligenin
        2) Specific beta$_2$ stimulant
      b. Strength
        1) 90 mcg/inhalation
        2) 5 mg/ml
      c. Dosage
        1) Metered dose inhaler
        2) 1 to 2 inhalations every 4 to 6 hours
        3) 0.2 to 0.5 ml in 3 ml saline
      d. Hazards
        1) Minimal

B. Mucolytics
   1. Acetylcysteine (Mucomyst)
      a. Action
        1) Lowers viscosity of mucus by replacing disulfide bonds
      b. Strength
        1) 10%; 20%
        2) 100 mg/ml; 200 mg/ml
      c. Dosage
        1) 2 to 3 ml
      d. Hazards
        1) Bronchospasm
        2) Nausea
        3) Oral blisters

   2. Sodium bicarbonate
      a. Action
         1) Increases bronchial pH
      b. Strength
         1) 2%; 20 mg/ml
      c. Dosage
         1) 2 to 5 ml/nebulization
      d. Hazards
         1) Increased bronchial pH may produce irritation to the bronchial tree
C. Parasympatholytics
   1. Atropine sulfate
      a. Action
         1) Blocks cyclic GMP
         2) Inhibits activity of acetylcholine
      b. Strength
         1) 0.2% to 1.0%
      c. Dosage
         1) 0.3 to 1.0 mg in 3 ml saline
      d. Hazards
         1) Mucus plugging
         2) Tachycardia
         3) Thickening of secretions
D. Antiasthmatic
   1. Cromolyn sodium (Intal)
      a. Action
         1) Inhibits degranulation of mast cells
         2) Prevents the release of histamine, heparin and SRS-A
         3) Prophylactic agent

b. Strength
1) 20 mg capsules (powder)
2) 20 mg ampules (solution)
c. Dosage
1) One capsule in spin-haler 4 times daily
2) One ampule per nebulization
3) Drug must be inhaled to be absorbed
d. Hazards
1) Bronchospasm
2) Nasal congestion

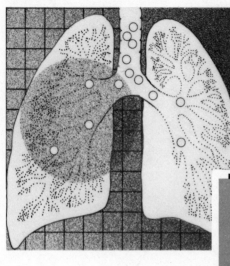

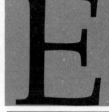

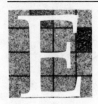

I. Electrocardiography

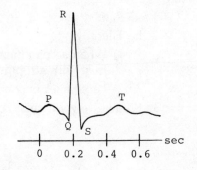

A. Interpretation
1. P wave—atrial depolarization
2. PR interval—beginning of P wave to the onset of ventricular depolarization
3. QRS complex—ventricular depolarization; atrial repolarization lost in complex
4. ST segment—end of ventricular depolarization; beginning of repolarization
5. T wave—ventricular repolarization

B. Rhythms

  1. Sinus tachycardia

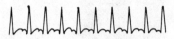

    a. Rate >100

    b. Therapy

      1) Treat underlying cause

  2. Sinus bradycardia

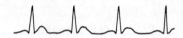

    a. Rate <60

    b. Therapy

      1) When accompanied with hypotension, treat with atropine

      2) Pacemaker may be indicated

  3. Premature ventricular contraction (PVC)

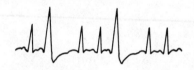

    a. Ventricular depolarization that happens before the next normal beat

      1) Unifocal—PVC span constant

      2) Multifocal—PVC span varies

    b. Bigeminy—every other beat is PVC

    c. Trigeminy—two normal beats plus one PVC, or one normal beat plus two PVCs

    d. Therapy

      1) Lidocaine

4. Ventricular fibrillation (V-fib)

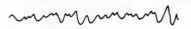

   a. No ventricular depolarization; no cardiac output
   b. Therapy
      1) For fine V-fib, give sodium bicarbonate before defibrillation
      2) For coarse V-fib, defibrillate immediately
5. Ventricular tachycardia (V-tach)

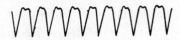

   a. Three or more ventricular beats occurring in succession at a rate >100
   b. Therapy
      1) Lidocaine
      2) If hemodynamically unstable give countershock
6. Atrial flutter

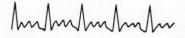

   a. Rapid and steady atrial depolarization
   b. P waves resemble sawtooth rhythm
   c. Atrial rate ranges between 220 and 350 beats per minute
   d. Therapy
      1) DC countershock
      2) Digitalis
      3) Quinidine

7. Atrial fibrillation

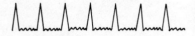

   a. Lack of atrial contraction
   b. Atrial rate varies between 400 to 700 beats per minute
   c. No P waves present
   d. Therapy
      1) Synchronized dc countershock
      2) Digitalis
      3) Quinidine
8. Atrioventricular block
   a. First degree block

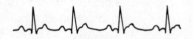

      1) Delay in passage of impulse
      2) Each P wave followed by QRS complex
      3) PR interval prolonged beyond 0.2 sec
   b. Second degree block

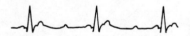

      1) Some impulses conducted; some blocked
      2) Classification
         a) Type I—Wenckebach
            (1) Increasingly prolonged PR intervals with dropped QRS complex
         b) Type II—Mobitz II
            (1) PR interval normal or prolonged, but constant

(2) Wide QRS complex
c. Third degree block

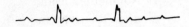

1) Complete lack of ventricular and atrial conduction
2) Varying PR interval
d. Therapy
1) Atropine
2) Pacemaker

C. Conditions that create abnormal EKG waves
1. Myocardial infarction
   a. Abnormal Q-waves
   b. T inversion
2. Mitral stenosis
   a. Notched P-wave
3. Hypokalemia
   a. Presence of U waves
   b. Depressed T-waves
4. Hypocalcemia
   a. Prolonged ST-segment
5. Hypercalcemia
   a. Shortened ST-segment
   b. QRS prolongation
6. Hyperkalemia
   a. ST depression
   b. Tall, peaked T-waves

D. Leads
1. Standard leads
   a. I—left arm (+); right arm (−)

    b. II—left leg (+); right arm (−)

    c. III—left leg (+); left arm (−)

2. Augmented leads

    a. aVR—right arm (+); left arm and left leg (−)

    b. aVL—left arm (+); left leg and right arm (−)

    c. aVF—left leg (+); left arm and right arm (−)

3. Precordial leads

    a. V_1—fourth intercostal space, right sternal border

    b. V_2—fourth intercostal space, left sternal border

    c. V_3—midway between V_2 and V_4

    d. V_4—5th intercostal space, midclavicular line

    e. V_5—same level as V_4, anterior axillary line

    f. V_6—same level as V_5, midaxillary line

    g. V_7—same level as V_6, posterior axillary line

    h. V_8—same level as V_7, midscapular line

E. ECG graph

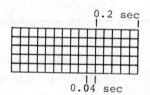

1. Normal paper speed 25 mm/sec

2. Vertical lines

    a. 1 mm = 0.04 sec (small boxes)

    b. 5 mm = 0.2 sec (large boxes)

3. Calculating rate

    a. Multiply number of boxes from the start of one wave to the beginning of the next same wave (example, P to P wave) by the specific mm/sec (1 mm/0.04 sec or 5 mm/0.2 sec)

b. Divide 60 sec by the number calculated above

II. Electrodes

A. PO_2 electrode—Clark

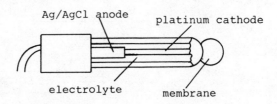

Ag/AgCl anode   platinum cathode

electrolyte   membrane

1. Polarographic principle
2. Measures oxygen by electron consumption
3. Silver/silver chloride anode; platinum cathode
4. Polypropylene membrane
   a. Blood/electrode barrier
   b. Promotes slow diffusion of oxygen molecules
5. Phosphate–potassium chloride electrolyte solution

B. CO_2 electrode—Severinghaus

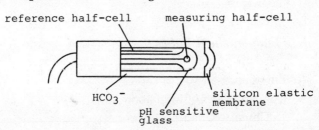

reference half-cell   measuring half-cell

HCO_3^- silicon elastic membrane

pH sensitive glass

1. Measures CO_2 by the change in H^+ concentration
   a. Proportional to the amount of CO_2 present
2. Modified pH electrode
3. Silicon elastic membrane
4. Bicarbonate electrolyte solution

C. pH electrode—Sanz

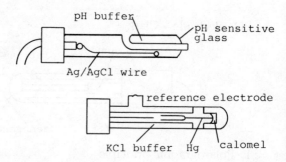

1. Potentiometric principle
2. Composed of two half-cells with a liquid junction
   a. Silver/silver chloride measuring electrode
   b. Mercury/mercurous chloride (calomel) reference electrode
   c. Half-cells connected by a potassium chloride salt bridge

III. Endotracheal Tubes

A. Emergency airway of choice
B. Complications of intubation
   1. Dental accidents

    2. Laryngospasm

    3. Right main stem intubation

    4. Esophageal intubation

C. Composition of tubes

    1. Polyvinyl chloride (PVC)

       a. Most common material

    2. Silastic (silicone)

       a. Used in pediatrics

       b. Low tissue toxicity

       c. Only few sizes have cuffs

    3. Nylon

    4. Teflon

D. Size of endotracheal tube internal diameter (ID) *versus* age of patient

Size ID (*mm*)	Patient
1. 2.5	premature infants
2. 3.0	newborn
3. 3.5	6 month old
4. 4.0–6.5	1–10 year old
5. 8.0–8.5 (±1 size)	adult female
6. 8.5–9.0 (±1 size)	adult male

E. Common sizes of endotracheal tubes with ID and OD

Size (*mm*)	ID	OD
1. 5	6	8
2. 6	7	10
3. 7	8	11
4. 8	9	12
5. 9	9.5	13

IV. Equations

A. Airway pressure

$$R_{aw} = \frac{\text{peak pressure (cm } H_2O) - \text{plateau pressure (cm } H_2O)}{\text{airflow (L/sec)}}$$

Peak pressure—pressure necessary to exceed airway resistance and compliance

Plateau pressure—pressure necessary to exceed compliance only

B. Alveolar air equation

$$P_AO_2 = (P_B - P_{H_2O})(F_IO_2) - PaCO_2(1.25)$$

C. Alveolar ventilation

$$\dot{V}_A = \dot{V}_E - \dot{V}_D = (V_t - V_D)f$$

D. A − aDO$_2$

$$P_AO_2 - PaO_2$$

E. Cardiac output (ml)

$$CO = \frac{\dot{V}O_2}{CaO_2 - CvO_2} \times 100$$

Normal $\dot{V}_{O_2}$ 250 L/min

Normal $CaO_2 - CvO_2$ 5 vol%

F. Arterial oxygen content (vol%)

$$CaO_2 = (1.34 \times Hb \times HbO_2 \text{ arterial}) + 0.003 \times PaO_2$$

Venous oxygen content (vol%)

$$CvO_2 = (1.34 \times Hb \times HbO_2 \text{ venous}) + 0.003 \times PvO_2$$

G. Compliance (L/cm H$_2$O)

$$C_T = 1/C_L + 1/C_{CW}$$

C_T = Total compliance (normal value 0.1 L/cm H$_2$O)

C_L = Lung compliance (normal value 0.2 L/cm H_2O)

C_{CW} = Chest wall compliance (normal value 0.2 L/cm H_2O)

$$\text{Dynamic compliance} = \frac{\text{mechanical Vt}}{\text{peak pressure} - \text{peep}}$$

Elastance = $1/C_L$

Specific compliance = C_L/FRC

✗ Static compliance = $\dfrac{\text{mechanical Vt}}{\text{plateau pressure} - \text{peep}}$

H. Deadspace (%)

$$V_D = \frac{PaCO_2 - PECO_2}{PaCO_2} \times Vt$$

I. Drug conversion

1 ml = 1 g

1 g = 1000 mg

1000 mg = 1 ml

Example: 0.1% = 1 g : 1000 ml = 1000 mg : 1000 ml
         = 1 mg : 1 ml

J. Drug dosage

$$\frac{\text{original strength}}{\text{known amount}} = \frac{\text{desired strength}}{\text{unknown amount}}$$

OR

$$\text{percentage strength (fraction)} = \frac{\text{solute (g or ml)}}{\text{total amount}}$$

K. Duration of cylinder usage

$$\frac{\text{psi reading} \times \text{cylinder factor}}{\text{LPM}}$$

L. Expected PaO_2 when $FIO_2 < 1.0$

$PaO_2 = (\%FIO_2 \times 7) - 50$

M. FiO_2

$$FiO_2 = \frac{x(0.21) + y}{x + y}$$

where x = air LPM

where y = O_2 LPM

Air to O_2 ratio

FiO_2 (%)	Air : O_2
24	25 : 1
28	10 : 1
35	5 : 1
40	3 : 1
50	1.7 : 1
60	1 : 1
70	0.6 : 1
100	0 : 1

N. Helium conversion

Helium Concentration	*Factor*
80% He + 20% O_2	1.8
70% He + 30% O_2	1.6

Actual flow = factor $\times$ indicated flow

O. Inspiratory time

It = Vt/$\dot{V}$ (L/sec)   OR   I(x) + E(x) = 60 sec/rate

Example: Vt = 800 ml   Example: Rate = 30

Peak flow = 40 LPM   I : E = 1 : 1.5

First change 40 LPM   1(x) + 1.5(x) = 60/30

to ml/sec   2.5(x) = 2

40 LPM = 667 ml/sec   x = 2/2.5

$\dfrac{800}{667}$ = 1.2 (inspiratory time)   x = 0.8 (inspiratory time)

P. Stroke volume

SV = CO (ml)/HR

CO = cardiac output

HR = heart rate

Q. Parameter change

$PaCO_2 \times f \times Vt = PaCO_2' \times f' \times Vt'$

Example: $PaCO_2 = 49$ mm Hg

$\qquad$ f = 10

$\qquad$ Vt = 0.8 L

Find new $PaCO_2$ (expected) when the rate is increased to 15

49 mm Hg $\times$ 10 $\times$ 0.8 L = (x) $\times$ 15 $\times$ 0.8 L

$392 = 12(x)$

$392/12 = x$

$32.6 = x =$ expected $PaCO_2$

R. Relative humidity

RH = AH/PH

AH = actual humidity (content)

PH = potential humidity (capacity)

Temperature	Potential Humidity
37°C	44 mg/L
21°C	18 mg/L

Humidity deficit = P_{H_2O} in alveolar air minus P_{H_2O} in inspired air

S. Mean arterial pressure

MAP = ⅓ (systolic − diastolic) + diastolic

T. Shunt

$Qs/Qt = CcO_2 - CaO_2/CcO_2 - CvO_2$

$CcO_2 = (P_AO_2 \times 0.003) + (1.34 \times Hb)$

Clinical calculation of shunt

$650 - PaO_2 \times (5/100)$

Where $F_IO_2 = 1.0$

Where $PaO_2 > 150$ mm Hg

U. Total flow

Example: Find the total flow of 0.4 FIO_2 with the flow-meter set at 6 LPM

0.4 = 3 : 1 (air : O_2 of 0.4)

3 + 1 = 4 (total flow at 1 LPM)

4 LPM × 6 LPM = 24 LPM
(total flow at 6 LPM)

V. *Esophageal Obturator*

A. Designed for intubation of the esophagus
B. Self-sealing mask
C. Precautions
    1. Never used in conscious patients
    2. Possible tracheal intubation
    3. Vomiting, aspiration upon removal
    4. Potential for gastric or esophageal rupture

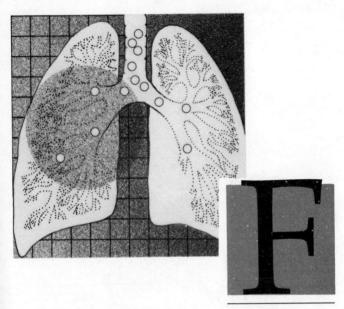

F

Flowmeters

Flow Patterns

Fluidics

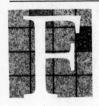

I. Flowmeters

A. Thorpe
  1. Regulates and indicates flow
  2. Compensated
     a. Indicated on label
     b. Ball jumps when
        plugged in
     c. Needle valve placed
        downstream
     d. Presence of back
        pressure; maintains
        accu-
        rate reading
  3. Noncompensated
     a. Needle valve placed upstream

Arrow indicates
gas flow

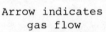
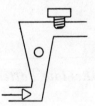

   b. Presence of back pressure; indicated flow is
      less than the patient is actually receiving

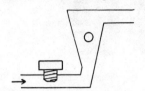

Arrow indicates gas flow

B. Bourdon gauge
   1. Calibrated to only indicate flow
   2. Actually measures pressure
   3. Presence of back pressure; gauge reads a higher
      flow than the patient is actually receiving

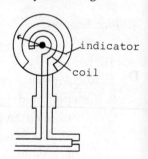

II. Flow Patterns

A. Square—Constant

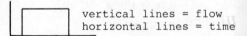

vertical lines = flow
horizontal lines = time

   1. Uninfluenced by changes in airway resistance
      and compliance

  2. Advantageous if the patient has an increased respiratory rate
  3. Ventilators with constant flow
     a. Ma-1
     b. Bourns Bear I and II
     c. Siemens Servo B and Servo C
B. Sine wave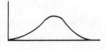
  1. Rotary-driven single circuit
  2. Reduces airway turbulence
  3. Ventilator with sine wave
     a. Emerson
C. Increasing flow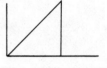
  1. Rotary-driven double circuit
  2. Causes a greater increase of intrathoracic pressures
  3. Ventilator with increasing flow
     a. Engstrom
D. Decreasing flow—Tapered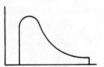
  1. Never tapers to zero
  2. Flow highest at the beginning of inspiration
  3. Equipment with decreasing flow
     a. Bennett PR-2
     b. Bird Mark 7 on air mix

III. Fluidics

A. Unites innate logic with gas flow
B. Requires no moving parts

C. Changes in gas flow incorporated by amplification
D. Coanda effect
   1. Changes the direction of gas flow by the application of subatmospheric pressure at the wall
E. Fluidic equipment
   1. Monaghan 225
   2. Sechrist—PEEP attachment
F. Correct operation is not altered by changes in atmosphere, temperature, or humidity
G. Types
   1. Flip-flop

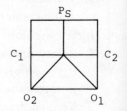

   2. AND/NAND

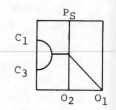

   3. OR/NOR

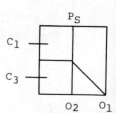

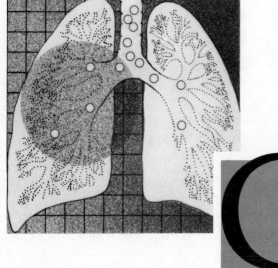

G

Gas Analyzers

Gas Laws

Gas Therapy

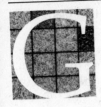

I. Gas Analyzers

A. Giesler tube
1. Measures nitrogen by ionizing a gas sample between a set of electrodes; a light is emitted that is proportional to the amount of nitrogen present
2. Pulmonary tests that use a Giesler tube analyzer
   a. 7 min N_2 washout
   b. Single breath N_2
B. Thermal conductivity
1. Measures He by generating a difference in heat from glass-coated thermistor beads connected to a wheatstone bridge circuit; the heat conducted away from the thermistors is proportional to the amount of He present
2. Pulmonary tests that use a thermal-conductivity analyzer
   a. Closed-circuit He dilution

C. Infrared absorption
   1. Measures CO_2 and CO contained in a gas sample
   2. Contains infrared beams that pass through parallel cells connected to an oscillating diaphragm; when a sample gas is introduced, the degree of oscillation is proportional to the CO_2 or CO present
   3. Pulmonary tests that use an infrared-absorption analyzer
      a. DL_{CO}

II. Gas Laws

A. Bohr effect
   1. At the tissue level, CO_2 diffused into the bloodstream heightens the release of O_2
B. Bohr equation
   1. $V_D/V_T = PaCO_2 - PECO_2/PaCO_2$
C. Boyle's law
   1. Temperature constant: $V_1P_1 = V_2P_2$
D. Charles' law
   1. Pressure constant: $V_1/T_1 = V_2/T_2$
E. Dalton's law
   1. The sum of the partial pressures in a gas is equal to the total pressure
F. Gay–Lussac's law
   1. Volume constant: $P_1/T_1 = P_2/T_2$

G. Graham's law

    1. Diffusion of a gas is indirectly proportional to the square root of its gram molecular weight (heavier molecules diffuse slower)

H. Haldane effect

    1. At the lung level, O_2 into the bloodstream heightens the release of CO_2

I. Henry's law

    1. Partial pressure gradient determines the amount of gas diffused

J. Universal law

    1. $V_1P_1/T_1 = V_2P_2/T_2$

III. Gas Therapy

A. Cylinder color code

Gas	Color Code
1. Oxygen	green/white
2. Carbon dioxide	gray
3. Nitrous oxide	light blue
4. Cyclopropane	orange
5. Helium	brown
6. Ethylene	red
7. Air	yellow/black

B. Cylinder markings

    1. Front

        a. DOT (Department of Transportation)

        b. Serial number

        c. Ownership

        d. Inspector symbol

   2. Back
      a. Manufacturer's mark
      b. Test date
      c. Elastic expansion values
      d. Hydrostatic test symbol
      e. Retest date
      f. Plant identification symbol
C. Cylinder testing
   1. Regulated by DOT
   2. Determines elastic expansion
   3. Cylinder retested every 5 to 10 yr
   4. Tested to a pressure of ⅚ of service pressure
D. Valve outlet connections
   1. ASS—American Standard System
      a. Cylinders above size E; flush threaded connections
      b. Holds <1500 psi
   2. PISS—Pin Index Safety System
      a. E cylinders and below
      b. Pin and hole connection; yoke type
      c. Holds >1500 psi
      d. Gas connection positions

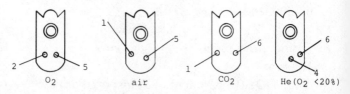

   3. DISS—Diameter Index Safety System
      a. Low-pressure system; thread connections
      b. Holds <200 psi

E. Pop-off valves
  1. Large cylinders
     a. Frangible disc
        1) Ruptures at pressures within 5% of cylinder bursting pressure
  2. Small cylinders
     a. Fusible plug
        1) Melts at temperature of 77°C
F. Cylinder factors and cubic foot capacities

Cylinder size	Factor (L/psi)	Cubic foot (cu ft)
1. D	0.16	12.7
2. E	0.28	22
3. G	2.41	187
4. H	3.14	244

G. Duration of flow

  1. Equation: $\dfrac{\text{psi reading} \times \text{factor}}{\text{LPM}}$

  2. Patient safety factor
     a. Subtract 500 psi from the gauge reading of E cylinders and below
     b. Subtract 300 psi from the gauge reading on cylinders larger than E

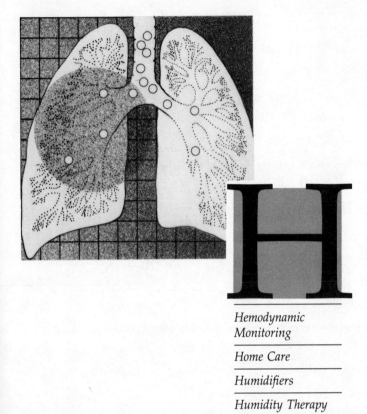

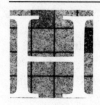

I. Hemodynamic Monitoring

A. Indications
  1. Heart failure
     a. Evaluation of proper drug therapy and dosage
     b. Measurement of pulmonary capillary wedge pressure (PCWP) to evaluate left ventricular function
  2. Hypovolemia
     a. Measurement of PCWP to evaluate proper fluid replacement level (fluid challenge)
  3. ARDS
     a. Avoidance of overhydration using PCWP
     b. High mechanical peak inspiratory pressures are generated that compromise cardiac performance (especially with PEEP therapy)
        1) Swan-Ganz measurements provide a basis for evaluating the degree of cardiac impairment
     c. Determination of optimal PEEP level using the cardiac output measurement

    d. Assessment of the PCWP in patients with pulmonary edema

  4. Acute burn patients

    a. Monitoring PCWP for proper hydration levels

    b. Possible pulmonary edema or ARDS complication

  5. Renal failure

    a. The kidneys function to maintain the body's sodium and water levels

    b. In renal failure there is sodium retention (with edema) and water retention (with hypervolemia)

    c. Monitoring the PCWP can evaluate the severity and the course of therapy

B. Precautions

  1. Thrombus formation

  2. Recurrent sepsis

  3. Pulmonary hemorrhage

  4. Balloon rupture

C. Measurements

  1. Right atrium (RA)

    a. Normal value -1 to $+7$ mm Hg

    b. Reduced right atrial blood volume creates a decreased pressure

      1) Hypovolemia

      2) Hemorrhage

      3) Vasodilation

    c. Increased blood volume entering the right atrium creates an increased pressure

      1) Hypervolemia

2. Right ventricle (RV)
   a. Normal value 15 to 25/0 to 8 mm Hg
3. Pulmonary artery pressure (PAP)
   a. Normal value 15 to 25/8 to 15 mm Hg
   b. Reduced blood volume creates a decreased pressure
      1) Hypovolemia
      2) Hemorrhage
   c. Increased pulmonary vascular resistance (increased back pressure in the pulmonary vascular system backing to the pulmonary artery) creates an increased pressure
      1) Chronic obstructive pulmonary disease (COPD)
      2) Pulmonary emboli
      3) Pulmonary hypertension
      4) Hypoxia
      5) Right heart failure
4. Pulmonary capillary wedge pressure (PCWP)
   a. Normal value 6 to 12 mm Hg
   b. Decreased perfusion or reduced blood volume (low resistance) will create a decreased pressure
      1) Hypovolemia
      2) Pulmonary emboli
      3) Vasodilation
   c. Increased blood volume or increased resistance (back pressure, congestion) or heart failure will create an increased pressure
      1) Left heart failure
      2) Hypervolemia

3) Pulmonary edema
4) Fluid overload
d. Assesses left atrial pressure; left ventricular diastolic pressure
e. Measured under no flow conditions
5. Wave forms

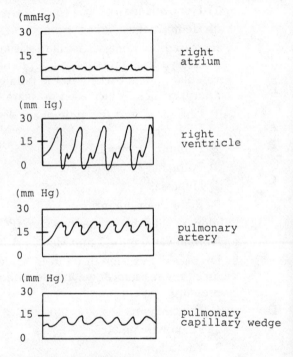

6. Examples of abnormal pressures
    a. Increased PAP; normal or decreased PCWP
        1) Pulmonary emboli
    b. Normal PAP; increased PCWP
        1) Left heart failure
    c. Increased PAP; normal PCWP

        1) Right heart failure

        2) Cor pulmonale

        3) Right to left shunt

    d. Increased PAP; increased PCWP

        1) Acute myocardial infarction

7. Ventilator management

    a. Record pressure readings at end exhalation

    b. PEEP therapy will increase PCWP reading

II. Home Care

A. Patient education of disease state essential

B. Oxygen therapy and administering of medications carefully explained for hazards and precautions

C. Equipment cleaning instructions

    1. Wash parts in mild detergent; rinse well

    2. Soak parts in vinegar solution for 20 min

    3. Rinse well

    4. Drain dry

    5. When dry, reassemble; store in clean plastic bags

D. Appropriate follow-up care or outpatient appointment

III. Humidifiers

A. Pass over (blow by)

    1. Gas passes over water surface

    2. Low efficiency

B. Bubble (diffusion)
1. Most common unit
2. Gas guided to below water surface
3. Increasing flow rates decrease efficiency

C. Jet
1. Produces aerosol
2. Water level less of an influence for efficiency

D. Bennett cascade (heated)
1. Advanced bubble type
2. Most commonly used with ventilators
3. 100% relative humidity provided
    a. Factors affecting humidity content
        1) Setting of heater
        2) Temperature of room
        3) Air flow
        4) Water level
        5) Length of wide-bore tubing
4. Some of the ventilator V_t may be lost due to the yielding of pressure of the cascade if not kept full

IV. Humidity Therapy

A. Indications
1. Intubated patients—upper airway bypassed
2. Patients receiving >30% oxygen therapy

B. Precautions
1. Asthmatics
2. Fluid overload patients
3. Edema

C. Relative humidity
1. RH = content/capacity
2. At 37°C, 100% RH = 44 mg/L
3. At 21°C, 100% RH = 18 mg/L
4. Cool saturated air causes a decreased RH when heated

D. Humidity deficit
1. P_{H_2O} in alveolar air minus inspired P_{H_2O}
2. 44 mg/L minus actual humidity

E. Complications of inadequate humidification
1. Atelectasis
2. Pneumonia
3. Bacterial infiltration
4. Tenacious secretions

V. Hypoxemia

A. Etiology
1. Decreased alveolar oxygen tension
   a. Responds to oxygen therapy
2. Shunting
   a. Does not respond to oxygen therapy

B. Physiologic effects
1. Tachycardia—primary sign of hypoxemia
2. Increased ventilation
3. Increased cardiac output
4. Decreased blood pressure

C. Classification
1. Mild—PaO_2 60 to 80 mm Hg

    2. Moderate—PaO_2 40 to 60 mm Hg

    3. Severe—PaO_2 < 40 mm Hg

D. Classification with supplemental oxygen

    1. Uncorrected—PaO_2 < 60 mm Hg

    2. Corrected—PaO_2 60 to 100 mm Hg

    3. Overcorrected—PaO_2 > 100 mm Hg

VI. *Hypoxia*

A. Anemic hypoxia

    1. Reduced holding capacity for oxygen

    2. Absolute anemia

       a. Decreased hemoglobin level

       b. Treat with packed red blood cells

    3. Relative anemia

       a. Normal hemoglobin level

       b. Complication of carbon monoxide poisoning

         1) Treat with 100% nonrebreathing mask

         2) Hyperbaric oxygen

    4. Usually does not show hypoxemia or cyanosis

       a. Normal PaO_2 levels

B. Histotoxic hypoxia

    1. Inability of oxygen to be released from hemo-globin at the tissue level

    2. Complication of cyanide poisoning

    3. Usually does not show hypoxemia or cyanosis

       a. Normal PaO_2 levels

C. Stagnant (circulatory) hypoxia

    1. Reduced cardiac output with slow blood flow

2. Vasoconstriction a cause of
3. Treatment aimed at increasing cardiac output with heart medications
D. Hypoxemic hypoxia
   1. Reduced oxygen diffusion
   2. Major causes are shunting and V/Q mismatch

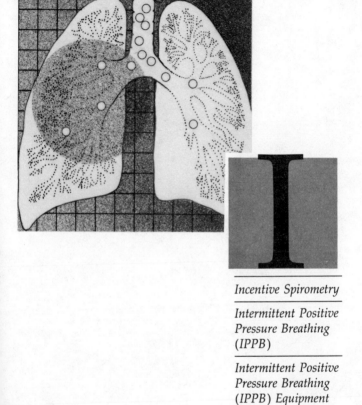

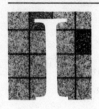

I. Incentive Spirometry

A. Maximum sustained inspiration
B. Prophylactic therapy to reduce the incidence of atelectasis and retained secretions
C. Goals
   1. To optimally inflate the lungs
   2. To promote effective coughing measures
   3. To observe for early pneumonia or atelectasis
D. Hazards
   1. Hyperventilation
   2. Paresthesia

II. Intermittent Positive Pressure Breathing (IPPB)

A. Indications
   1. FVC < 15 ml/kg
   2. Patient unable to cough or deep breathe

B. Goals
  1. To improve ventilation
  2. To promote the cough
  3. To deliver medication
C. Administering an effective treatment
  1. Slow, deep breaths; 7 to 10 per min
  2. Inspiratory time of 2 to 4 sec
  3. Inspiratory pause
  4. Expiratory time of 2 to 4 sec
  5. Delivering 75% of the patient's limited vital capacity
D. Physiologic effects
  1. Decreased work of breathing during the treatment
  2. Increased tidal volumes
  3. Improved ventilatory cycle (I : E ratio)
  4. Bronchodilation
E. Hazards
  1. Hyperventilation
  2. Hyperoxygenation
  3. Increased air trapping
     a. Forcing air in but not out
  4. Applied positive pressure
     a. Decreased cardiac output
     b. Decreased venous return
     c. Increased intracranial pressure
     d. Pneumothorax
     e. Hypotension
F. Contraindication
  1. Tension pneumothorax

III. *Intermittent Positive Pressure Breathing (IPPB) Equipment*

A. Bennett PR-2
1. Classification
   a. Pressure   positive
   b. Power   pneumatic
   c. Modes   assist, assist/control
   d. Cycling   flow, time
   e. Limit   pressure, low terminal flow
   f. Flow pattern   decaying
2. Use of expiratory nebulizer adds to patient's exhaled volumes
3. Terminal flow
   a. Allows flow to decrease to a level low enough to close Bennett valve
   b. Used when minor leaks are present—mask treatments
   c. Dilutes source gas
4. Built-in I:E ratio of 1:1.5
5. Diluter
   a. Pushed in; air mix
   b. Pulled out; 100% source gas
6. Peak flow
   a. Full open; maximum flow
   b. Decreased; flow rate 15 LPM
   c. Not a flow rate control like the Bird Mark series
7. Expiratory time control
   a. Decreases gas flow
   b. Increases exhalation time

    8. Rate

      a. Allows adjustable I : E ratios

B. PR-1

    1. Differences from PR-2

      a. No expiratory time control

      b. No peak flow control

      c. No terminal flow

      d. Incorporates a continuous nebulizer

C. Bird Mark 7

    1. Classification

a. Pressure	positive
b. Power	pneumatic
c. Modes	assist, assist/control
d. Cycling	pressure
e. Limit	flow
f. Flow pattern	decaying with air mix square with 100% source gas

    2. Magnetism *versus* gas pressure

      a. Primary principle of operation

    3. Pneumatic clutching

      a. As pressure builds in the right chamber, the venturi gate closes; incoming gas then exits through entrainment ports to the left (ambient) chamber

      b. On the next breath, this source gas is entrained through the venturi; patient receives increased oxygen concentration (60% to 90%)

    4. Diluter

      a. Pushed in; 100% source gas

        1) Square wave

        2) 0 to 50 LPM flow

      b. Pulled out; air mix
        1) Decaying wave
        2) 0 to 80 LPM flow
  5. Expiratory timer
      a. Time cycled
      b. Greater leak; decreased exhalation time; increased rate
  6. Flow rate control
      a. Increased oriface size; increased nebulization
      b. Flow rate limited to 0 to 50 LPM with 100% source gas
  7. Pressure and sensitivity settings
      a. Adjusts the position of each magnet
      b. The closer the magnet is to the plate, the stronger the force needed to overcome the resistance

D. Bird Mark 8
  1. Same as the Bird Mark 7
  2. Incorporates negative end expiratory pressure (NEEP)
      a. Need to adjust the sensitivity when in use

E. Bird Mark 9
  1. Same as the Bird Mark 8
  2. Provides pressures up to 200 cm H_2O
  3. Double-jet venturi system
      a. Provides high flow rates
  4. Used for veterinary medicine

F. Bird Mark 10
  1. Same as the Bird Mark 7
  2. Permanently set on air mix
  3. Inspiratory flow accelerator added
      a. Leak compensation

IV. *Intrapleural Pressure*

A. Pressure gradient between the pleural space and lung
B. Normal value at FRC −4 cm H_2O
C. Inspiration; drops to −9 cm H_2O
D. Expiration; returns to −4 cm H_2O
E. Greater negative value at apex (−10 cm H_2O) than base (−2 cm H_2O)
  1. Gravity dependent
  2. Bases easier to inflate and ventilate

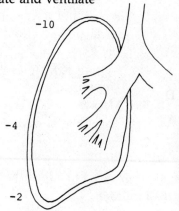

V. *Isolation Techniques*

A. Respiratory isolation
  1. Pathogens—droplets from the respiratory tract
    a. Active tuberculosis
    b. Pertussis
    c. Pneumonia—*Staphylococcus aureus*

   2. Masks required
   3. Gowns required when holding infants
   4. Gloves not needed

B. Enteric isolation
   1. Pathogens transmitted in feces
   2. Masks not required
   3. Gloves and gown required when handling fecal material

C. Wound and skin isolation
   1. Pathogens found in wounds, dressings, linens
   2. Gowns worn, in some cases gloves must be worn
   3. Masks worn for respiratory precaution

D. Blood isolation
   1. Blood pathogens
      a. Malaria
      b. Serum hepatitis
   2. Masks not necessary
   3. Gloves and gown worn for precaution

E. Strict isolation
   1. Pathogens spread by contact or air
   2. All highly communicable diseases
      a. Diphtheria
      b. Smallpox
      c. Rabies
      d. Acquired immunodeficiency syndrome (AIDS)
   3. Masks, gowns, and gloves are all required

F. Protective isolation (reverse)
1. Protects uninfected patient who has a lowered immune system
    a. Cancer therapy
    b. Leukemia
    c. Patients on immunosuppressive drugs
2. Masks, gowns, and gloves are all required

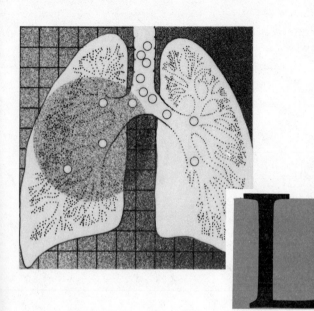

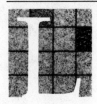

I. Loops: Flow Volume Curves

A. Normal

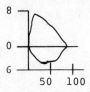

Vertical lines:
Flow (L/sec)
Horizontal lines:
Volume (% FVC)

B. Obstructive (COPD)

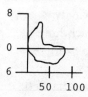

C. Restrictive

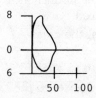

109

D. Early airway closure

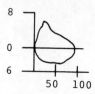

E. Large airway obstruction

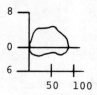

II. *Lung Anatomy*

A. Left and right lungs separated by the mediastinum
B. Parietal pleura—lines each thoracic cavity
C. Visceral pleura—membrane lining each lung
D. Intrapleural space—potential space existing between the parietal and visceral pleura
E. Hilus—only area where the lungs are attached
F. Lung subdivisions and generations
   1. With each branching of the tracheobronchial tree, a new generation is produced
   2. With each successive generation, the cross-sectional area greatly increases
   3. Conducting zone (generations #0 to #15)
      a. Functions to conduct inspired gases to the respiratory zone

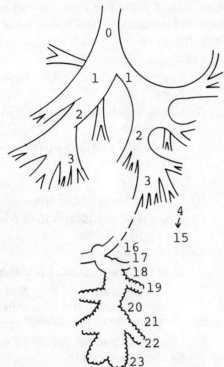

numbers represent each generation
see text that follows

    b. Contains no alveoli; does not participate in
       gas exchange
    c. Composes the anatomic deadspace; volume
       is approximately 150 ml
    d. Nose
       1) Contains cartilage and bone
       2) Has two external openings—nostrils
          (nares)

3) Each nostril is divided by the septal cartilage and contains a nasal fossae (cavity) with three regions
   a) Vestibular region
      (1) Contains vibrissae (coarse nasal hairs)
      (2) Contains sebaceous glands that secrete sebum
      (3) Lined with stratified squamous epithelium
   b) Olfactory region
      (1) Contains the sense of smell
      (2) Lined with pseudostratified columnar epithelial cells
   c) Respiratory region
      (1) Contains the turbinates (conchae)
         (a) Creates turbulent flow that filters, heats, and humidifies (up to 80%) the inspired gases
      (2) Lined with pseudostratified ciliated columnar epithelium
4) The nose ends at the nasopharynx
e. Pharynx
   1) Produces phonation by changing its shape
   2) Nasopharynx
      a) Lined with pseudostratified ciliated columnar epithelium
   3) Oropharynx
      a) Lined with stratified squamous epithelium

   4) Laryngopharynx (hypopharynx)
      a) Lined with stratified squamous epithelium
      b) Leads to the larynx (anteriorly) and to the esophagus (posteriorly)
f. Larynx
   1) Connects the upper airway to the lower airway
   2) Opening of the larynx—glottis
      a) Narrowest part of the upper airway in the adult
   3) Major cartilages contained within
      a) Thyroid cartilage (Adam's apple)
      b) Cricoid cartilage
         (1) Narrowest part of the upper airway in infants and small children
      c) Cricothyroid membrane
         (1) Connects the thyroid and cricoid cartilages
         (2) Lies below the level of the vocal cords
         (3) Emergency airway puncture site (cricothyroidotomy)
      d) Arytenoid cartilage
         (1) Produces vocal cord movement
      e) Epiglottis
         (1) Attaches to the thyroid cartilage
         (2) Functions to guard the glottis during swallowing
   4) Lined with stratified squamous epithelium above the vocal cords and pseudo-

stratified columnar epithelium below the
vocal cords

5) Larynx is divided into sections by the
ventricular folds (false vocal cords) and
the vocal folds (true vocal cords)

g. Trachea (generation #0)

1) Extends from the cricoid cartilage to the
carina

2) Contains 16 to 20 C-shaped cartilagenous
rings that open posteriorly

3) 11 to 13 cm in length

4) The trachea and larger airways are composed of three major layers

a) Epithelial lining

(1) Pseudostratified ciliated columnar
epithelium

(2) Contains mucous and serous
glands along with cilia

b) Lamina propria (submucosa)

(1) Contains fibrous tissue with small
blood vessels, lymphatic vessels,
and nerves

c) Cartilagenous layer

(1) Contains a varying amount of cartilage that becomes absent in tubes
less than 1 mm in diameter

5) Cross-sectional area of the trachea is approximately 2.5 cm^2

h. Mainstem bronchi—primary bronchi (generation #1)

1) Bifurcates at the carina

2) Has two main units

3) Right mainstem bronchus
   a) Forms a 25° angle from the midline of the trachea
   b) Approximately 2.5 cm in length
   c) Approximately 1.4 cm in diameter
   d) Aspirated bodies are commonly lodged in the right mainstem bronchus due to its angle from the trachea and its larger diameter compared with the left mainstem bronchus
4) Left mainstem bronchus
   a) Forms a 40° to 60° angle from the midline of the trachea
   b) Approximately 5 cm in length
   c) Approximately 1.0 cm in diameter

i. Lobar bronchi—secondary bronchi (generation #2)
   1) The right and left mainstem bronchi branch to form five lobar bronchi
   2) The right mainstem bronchus branches to form three lobar bronchi
      a) Right upper lobar (RUL)
      b) Right middle lobar (RML)
      c) Right lower lobar (RLL)
   3) The left mainstem bronchus branches to form two lobar bronchi
      a) Left upper lobar (LUL)
         (1) Includes the left lingula
      b) Left lower lobar (LLL)

j. Segmental bronchi—tertiary bronchi (generation #3)

1) The five lobar bronchi branch into a total of 18 segments
   a) Right upper lobar bronchus
      (1) Anterior segment
      (2) Apical segment
      (3) Posterior segment
   b) Right middle lobar bronchus
      (1) Lateral segment
      (2) Medial segment
   c) Right lower lobar bronchus
      (1) Medial basilar segment
      (2) Anterior basilar segment
      (3) Lateral basilar segment
      (4) Superior basilar segment
      (5) Posterior basilar segment
   d) Left upper lobar bronchus
      (1) Apical–posterior segment
      (2) Anterior segment
      (3) Lingula section
         (a) Superior segment
         (b) Inferior segment
   e) Left lower lobar bronchus
      (1) Anteromedial basilar segment
      (2) Lateral basilar segment
      (3) Superior basilar segment
      (4) Posterior basilar segment

2) The superior and posterior basilar segments show an increased occurrence of atelectasis and pneumonia in bedridden patients owing to the supine position of

the patient and the segment's posterior branching

3) The cartilagenous rings contained within these segments become irregular in size and shape as compared with the mainstem bronchi and lobar bronchi

4) Pseudostratified ciliated columnar epithelium line each segment

k. Small bronchi—subsegmental (generations #4 to #9)

1) Diameter of these bronchi is approximately 1 mm to 6 mm

2) Cartilagenous rings give way to cartilagenous plaques by the ninth generation

3) Pseudostratified ciliated columnar epithelium lines the subsegmental bronchi

4) Contains up to 2000 units

4. Transitional zone

a. Bronchioles (generations #10 to #15)

1) Diameter is less than 1 mm

2) No cartilage is present

3) Airway patency relies on the fibrous, elastic, and smooth muscle tissues that are present

4) Lined with pseudostratified ciliated cuboidal epithelium

5) Contains up to 4000 units

b. Terminal bronchioles (generation #16)

1) Diameter is approximately 0.5 mm

2) Smallest airway without alveoli

3) Epithelial cells change from cuboidal to flattened cuboidal

4) Cilia and submucosal gland are absent
5) Clara cells become prominent
   a) Partly responsible for surfactant production
6) Contain 65,000 to 130,000 units
7) Total cross-sectional area is approximately 180 cm^2

5. Respiratory zone
  a. Respiratory bronchioles (generations #17 to #19)
    1) At this level, the lung parenchyma begins
    2) Diameter averages 0.4 mm
    3) Scattered areas of alveoli are present
    4) Flattened cuboidal epithelium are present along with simple squamous epithelium (from the scattered alveoli)
    5) Contains up to 500,000 units
  b. Alveolar ducts (generations #20 to #22)
    1) Walls of the alveolar ducts are composed entirely of alveoli
    2) Alveolar ducts may give rise to a single alveoli or to alveolar sacs, which contain two or more alveoli
    3) Lined with simple squamous epithelium (alveolar epithelium)
    4) Alveoli attached to alveolar ducts participate in approximately 35% of alveolar gas exchange
    5) Contains approximately 1 million to 4 million units
  c. Alveolar sacs (generation #23)
    1) Last unit in the generation numbers

      2) Found in clusters (15 to 20 sacs) with common septal walls

      3) Collateral circulation is present because of the pores of Kohn (small holes present in the alveolar walls)

      4) Contains approximately 8 million units

      5) Cross-sectional area is approximately 11,800 cm^2

d. Alveoli

      1) Air spaces where gas exchange occurs

      2) Approximately 300 million alveoli are present in the adult

      3) 15 to 25 million alveoli are present at birth

e. Alveolar capillary membrane

      1) Thickness of the membrane is approximately 0.35 μ to 1.0 μ

      2) Alveolar cell types

         a) Type I alveolar cell

            (1) Squamous pneumocyte

            (2) Composes 95% of the alveolar surface

         b) Type II alveolar cell

            (1) Granular pneumocyte

            (2) Produces surfactant (lowers the surface tension of the alveolar lining)

         c) Type III alveolar cell

            (1) Alveolar macrophage

            (2) Injests incoming foreign material

      3) Alveolar capillary blood transit time is approximately 0.75 sec (see Pulmonary Blood Flow)

III. Lung Capacities

A. Total lung capacity (TLC)
   1. Maximum volume of gas the lung can hold during a full inspiration
   2. Normal value 6 L
B. Inspiratory capacity (IC)
   1. Maximum volume of air that can be inhaled from a resting expiratory level (FRC)
   2. Comprises 60% of the TLC
   3. Normally decreased with hyperventilation
   4. Normal value 3.6 L
C. Functional residual capacity (FRC)
   1. Volume of gas remaining in the lungs at the end of a spontaneous expiration—resting level
   2. Composed of expiratory reserve volume (ERV) plus residual volume (RV)
   3. Comprises 40% of the TLC
   4. Normal value 2.5 L
D. Vital capacity (VC)
   1. Maximum volume of gas that can be exhaled from a full inspiration
   2. Contains all lung volumes except RV
   3. Comprises 75% of the TLC
   4. Normal value 4.5 L

IV. Lung Volumes

A. Tidal volume (V_t)
   1. Volume added to and removed with each normal breath
   2. Normal value 500 ml

B. Expiratory reserve volume (ERV)
   1. At FRC, gas expired maximally
   2. Comprises 15% of the TLC
   3. Normal value 1 L
C. Residual volume (RV)
   1. Volume of air remaining in the lungs after a complete forced expiration
   2. Comprises 25% of the TLC
   3. Increased value normally seen with increased FRCs
   4. Normal value 1.5 L
D. Inspiratory reserve volume (IRV)
   1. Maximum inhalation after a resting inspiration
   2. Comprises 50% of the TLC
   3. Normal value 3.1 L

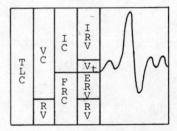

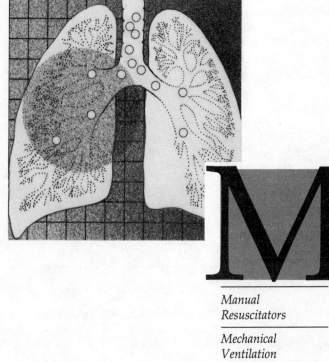

M

123

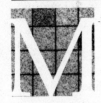

I. Manual Resuscitators

A. Guidelines
1. Must deliver 60% to 100% oxygen concentrations
2. No valve jamming during high air flows
3. No rebreathing
4. Attached reservoir
5. Self-refilling
   a. Can increase oxygen concentration if bag's refill time is restricted
B. Patient connections
1. 22 mm OD—anesthesia attachment
2. 15 mm ID—endotracheal or tracheal attachment

II. Mechanical Ventilation Classification

A. Positive pressure *versus* negative pressure
1. Positive pressure ventilators generate above atmospheric pressures to deliver inspiratory pressures

2. Negative pressure ventilators generate subatmospheric pressures on the lung to deliver inspiration

B. Flow generators
1. Constant flow generators
   a. Flow rate remains constant while inspiratory pressures vary
   b. Maintains a high source pressure to generate a gradient between the ventilator and patient
   c. Airway resistance and lung compliance does not affect gas delivery
   d. Incorporates a high internal resistance to guard the patient from the excessive pressure source
   e. Operating pressure must be kept well above the patient's peak inspiratory pressures
      1) As peak pressure approaches the operating pressure, the flow and pressure patterns change
      2) As a consequence, changing airway resistance and lung compliance will affect the delivery of gas
   f. Equipment
      1) BabyBird
      2) Bear I and Bear II
      3) Ma-1 and Ma-2
      4) Monaghan 225
      5) Ohio 560
      6) Sechrist
      7) Servo B and Servo C

2. Nonconstant flow generators
   a. Variable flow rate with constant flow pattern
   b. Changing lung compliance and airway resistance does not affect the flow pattern
   c. Equipment
      1) Bear I and Bear II
      2) Emerson IMV
      3) Ohio 550
      4) Servo B and Servo C
      5) Emerson 3-PV
C. Pressure generators
   1. Constant pressure ventilators
      a. Constant pressure given with varying tidal volumes
      b. Pressure is maintained with lung–thorax changes
      c. Operates with a low internal resistance
      d. Equipment
         1) Bear BP-200
         2) Gill-1
   2. Nonconstant pressure ventilator
      a. Variable pressures with a constant pressure pattern
      b. Changing lung–thorax conditions does not affect the pressure pattern
D. Time-cycled ventilators
   1. Inspiration is terminated at a present time interval
   2. Changes in airway resistance and lung compliance may give variable airway pressures and affect gas delivery

    3. Mainly used for neonates

    4. Equipment

      a. BabyBird

      b. Bear BP-200

      c. Monaghan 225

      d. Servo B and Servo C

E. Pressure-cycled ventilators

    1. Inspiration is terminated at a preset pressure

    2. Expiration is delayed if inflation hold is used

    3. Tidal volume and inspiratory time vary with airway resistance and lung compliance

    4. Mainly used for IPPB and home therapy

    5. Equipment

      a. Bird Mark series

      b. Monaghan 225

F. Volume-cycled ventilators

    1. Inspiration is terminated at a preset tidal volume

    2. Varying pressures are generated

    3. Most incorporate a pressure-limiting valve to prevent excessive delivered pressures

    4. Leaks in the system or patient may only be detected through exhaled tidal volume measurement

    5. Increased back pressure (decreased C_L) will cause part of the delivered tidal volume to be lost in the circuit by expansion on the tubing and compression in the humidifier, water traps

      a. Normal tubing compliance is approximately 3 ml/cm H_2O

      1) 3 ml of gas is lost in the circuit for each cm H_2O of peak pressure delivered

      2) If a patient is generating 30 cm H_2O peak pressure, 90 ml of the tidal volume will be lost to the circuit

      3) In severe restrictive diseases (ARDS, pulmonary fibrosis), more of the tidal volume is lost within the circuit owing to increasing peak pressures

G. Inspiratory cycle mechanism

  1. Parameter (when reached) that results in end inspiration

    a. Volume

    b. Time

    c. Flow

    d. Pressure

  2. Ventilators are classified by the parameter that ends inspiration

H. Inflation hold

  1. End inspiration is maintained to allow equal distribution of inspired gases

  2. Duration of hold is designated in 0 to 2 sec, or as a percentage of the total time of the ventilatory cycle

I. Expiratory retard

  1. Increases the resistance to exhalation

  2. A decrease in FRC is brought about by a more complete emptying of the lungs

  3. Used mainly in COPD patients who normally have an increased FRC

J. PEEP (see Positive End Expiratory Pressure (PEEP) Therapy)

K. Modes of ventilation

1. Control
   a. No active patient participation
   b. Indications
      1) Apneic patients
      2) CNS depression
2. Assist/Control
   a. Patient achieves ventilator tidal volumes with each breath; ventilator provides a back-up rate
   b. Can control hyperventilation by changing to an intermittent mandatory ventilation mode
3. Intermittent mandatory ventilation (IMV)
   a. Patient receives ventilator tidal volumes with a set rate; in addition, patient provides spontaneous tidal volumes
   b. Weaning technique
   c. Respiratory muscles kept active
   d. Useful with tachypneic patients
   e. Improves cardiovascular dynamics

III. Mechanical Ventilation Guidelines

A. Indications
1. Respiratory failure
2. Impending respiratory failure
3. Apnea
4. Oxygenation

B. Goal
  1. Maintain optimal cardiopulmonary status
C. Physiologic effects
  1. Increased mean airway pressure
  2. Increased deadspace (ventilation exceeding perfusion)
  3. Reduced cardiac output and venous return
  4. Decreased urine output
  5. Increased intracranial pressure (especially with PEEP therapy)
D. Initial settings
  1. V_t 10 to 15 ml/kg
  2. Rate 8 to 12 BPM
  3. I:E 1:2 in control mode
  4. Inspiratory time 0.5 to 2 sec
  5. Oxygen concentration determined by ABG analysis
  6. Appropriate peak flow to ensure adequate I:E ratio
     a. Increase peak flow to decrease inspiratory time
     b. Decrease peak flow to increase inspiratory time
E. Ventilator adjustments
  1. One parameter change with each ABG analysis
     a. Healthy lungs equilibrate after a parameter change in approximately 15 to 20 min
  2. Maintain PaO_2 60 to 100 mm Hg
     a. Oxygen concentration
     b. PEEP therapy
     c. ABG analysis

   3. Maintain eucapnic $PaCO_2$
     a. To decrease $PaCO_2$
       1) Increase V_t
       2) Increase rate
       3) Decrease deadspace
         a) Use only in control mode
     b. To increase $PaCO_2$
       1) Decrease V_t
       2) Decrease rate
       3) Increase deadspace
         a) Use only in control mode
   4. To correct an inverse I : E ratio
     a. Increase peak flow
     b. Decrease rate
     c. Decrease V_t
   5. Guidelines for decreasing oxygen concentration
     a. $PaO_2 > 300$ mm Hg
       1) Decrease FiO_2 0.2
     b. PaO_2 150 to 300 mm Hg
       1) Decrease FiO_2 0.1
     c. PaO_2 100 to 150 mm Hg
       1) Decrease FiO_2 0.05

F. Parameter guidelines for continued MV
   1. $Qs/Qt > 30\%$
   2. Spontaneous respiratory rate > 35
   3. Spontaneous $V_t < 4$ ml/kg
   4. VC < 15 ml/kg
   5. Negative inspiratory force (NIF) less than -20 cm H_2O
   6. $V_D/V_t > 60\%$

7. $PaO_2 < 50$ mm Hg with an $FIO_2 > 0.5$
8. $PaCO_2 > 55$ mm Hg
9. $pH < 7.25$
10. $A - aDO_2 > 350$ mm Hg
11. Minute ventilation > 10 LPM

IV. Mediastinum

A. A composite of organs and vessels that lie between the lungs
B. Organs and vessels composing the mediastinum
  1. Heart
  2. Ascending aorta
  3. Superior vena cavae
  4. Thoracic duct
  5. Esophagus
  6. Trachea
  7. Lymphatic structures
  8. Thymus gland
C. Mediastinal emphysema
  1. Presence of air within the mediastinum
  2. Common in neonates
  3. Complication of tracheostomy

V. Microbiology

A. Gram-negative rods
  1. *Pseudomonas aeruginosa*
     a. Found in the intestinal tract/skin of some individuals

b. Grows well in humidified environments
c. Commonly hospital-acquired
d. Cultured from sputum
   1) Foul smelling, tenacious, green
e. Causes pneumonia, septicemia, empyema
f. Treat with aminoglycosides

2. *Escherichia coli*
   a. Found in the intestinal tract
   b. Common nosocomial infection
   c. Causes septicemia, diarrhea, pneumonia
   d. Treat with gentamicin

3. *Haemophilus influenzae*
   a. Pfeiffer's bacillus
   b. Flora of the respiratory tract
   c. Common nosocomial infection
   d. Common cause of epiglottitis
   e. Cause of meningitis in children
   f. Treat with aminoglycosides

4. *Klebsiella pneumoniae*
   a. Friedlander's bacillus
   b. Flora of the nose, mouth
   c. Produces a red gelatinous sputum
   d. Causes pneumonia, lung abscess, septicemia
   e. Treat with gentamicin

B. Gram-positive rods
   1. *Clostridium perfingens*
      a. Causes gas gangrene
      b. Spore former

      c. Treat with hyperbaric oxygen, debridement, penicillin

  2. *Bacillus subtilis*

      a. Spore former

      b. Used as a biologic indicator for sterilization procedures

      c. Produces proteases—protein digesting enzymes

C. Gram-positive coccus

  1. *Staphylococcus aureus*

      a. Flora of the skin and respiratory tract

      b. Associated with food poisoning

      c. Causes pneumonia, empyema, septicemia

      d. Treat with tetracycline

  2. *Streptococcus pneumoniae*

      a. Exists in upper respiratory tract

      b. Surrounded by a capsule

      c. Usually acquired by respiratory droplets or contact

      d. Treat with penicillin, cephalosporin

  3. *Mycobacterium tuberculosis*

      a. Acid fast

      b. May enter body by inhalation of respiratory droplets

      c. Latent incubation period

      d. Treatment

         1) Streptomycin

         2) Rifampin

         3) Isoniazid

         4) Ethambutal

D. Staining properties
1. Acid fast (Ziehl-Neelsen)
   a. Mycobacterium species
   b. Positive test—stains red
2. Gram positive
   a. Positive test—stains blue, purple
3. Gram negative—stains red, pink

E. Viruses
1. Parainfluenza
   a. Major cause of croup
2. Respiratory syncytial virus
   a. Cause of infant bronchiolitis and pneumonia
3. Adenovirus
   a. Causes of upper and lower respiratory infections

F. Fungi
1. Types
   a. Yeast
   b. Molds
2. *Cryptococcosis neoformans*
   a. Most dangerous fungal disease
   b. Affects lungs and meninges
   c. Located in soil, pigeon droppings
   d. Enters body during inhalation
   e. Treat with amphotericin B
3. *Candida albicans*
   a. Most common fungi
   b. Found in intestine and vagina
   c. If mother is infected during pregnancy, it may cause thrush in newborn
   d. Treat with candicidin

4. *Histoplasma capsulatum*
    a. Summer flu
    b. Found in chicken coups, bat caves, dry dusty soil
    c. Contracted through inhalation
    d. Causes lung lesions and may spread to other organs
    e. Treat with amphotericin B
5. *Coccidioides immitis*
    a. Endemic to the southwest
    b. Common in people who work with the soil
    c. Infected by inhaling the spores
    d. Causes influenza-like infections

VI. Muscles of Ventilation

A. Diaphragm
    1. Innervated by 3 to 5 cervical roots
        a. Forms phrenic nerve
    2. Major muscle of ventilation
    3. Tidal volume excursion 1.5 cm
    4. Vital capacity excursion 10 cm
    5. During inspiration, diaphragm accounts for 75% of movement
B. Intercostal muscles
    1. Innervated by nerves from the spinal cord at T_1–T_{11}
    2. External intercostal muscles
        a. Moves ribs up and out during inspiration

b. Accounts for 25% of movement during inspiration

3. Internal intercostal muscles
   a. Pulls ribs down and in
   b. Used especially for forced expiration

C. Accessory muscles
   1. Scalene
   2. Sternocleidomastoid
   3. Trapezius
   4. Pectoralis

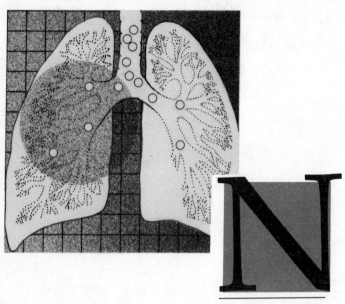

N

Nebulizers

Neonatal
Management

Neurotrauma

Nosocomial Infection

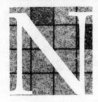

I. Nebulizers

A. Jet nebulizers
   1. Bernoulli's principle
      a. Increased velocity of a gas causes decreased lateral pressure resulting in increased forward pressure
   2. Employs baffles
      a. Reduces aerosol particle size
   3. Produces water content of 50 mg/L
   4. 55% of particles $< 10\ \mu$
B. Hydronamic nebulizer
   1. Hydrosphere (Babington)
   2. Contains a hollow glass sphere with holes at the top of the sphere that act as jets
   3. Negative pressure created by the jets pulls fluid around the sphere and into the gas flow
C. Classification
   1. Reservoir
      a. Mainstream

       1) Aerosol passes through gas flow
       2) Provides small aerosol particles with increased output
   b. Solution reservoir > 250 ml
   c. Provides continuous aerosol therapy
   d. Continuous heating element can provide 100% relative humidity
      1) Temperature factors
        a) Length of wide bore tubing
        b) Total flow
        c) Room temperature
        d) Solution level of reservoir
   e. Flow rate must exceed patient's inspiratory demand
  2. Intermittent reservoir
   a. Sidestream
      1) Aerosol passes into the flow of gas
      2) Provides small aerosol particles with decreased output
   b. Solution reservoir < 20 ml
   c. Indicated for delivery of medication

II. Neonatal Management

A. Fetal circulation
  1. Blood flows from the umbilical vein to the right atrium (RA)
   a. Umbilical blood contains highest blood PO_2
      1) Approximately 30 mm Hg
      2) 80% saturated

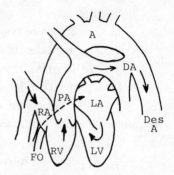

2. Blood then flows from the RA to the left atrium (LA) through the foramen ovale (FO)
3. Blood then enters the left ventricle (LV), then aorta (A) (perfuses head, upper body)
4. Returning blood from the upper body enters the RA, then flows to the right ventricle (RV) then through the pulmonary artery (PA)
5. PA blood then flows through the ductus arteriosis (DA) directly into the descending aorta (Des A) (perfuses lower body)
   a. Mixes with blood from the left ventricle

B. Apgar scoring
  1. Clinical evaluation after birth
     a. Heart rate
     b. Respiratory effort
     c. Muscle tone
     d. Color
     e. Reflex irritability
  2. Evaluation taken at 1 and 5 min after birth

     3. Scoring
       a. 0 to 2; severe respiratory distress
       b. 3 to 6; moderate distress
       c. 7 to 10; mild or no distress
     4. Heart rate score most important evaluation
       a. <100; suspected asphyxia

C. Silverman and Anderson index
     1. Index of respiratory distress
       a. Upper chest movement
       b. Lower chest movement
       c. Xyphoid retractions
       d. Nasal flaring
       e. Expiratory grunt
     2. Scoring
       a. 0; no respiratory distress
       b. 10; severe respiratory distress

D. Apnea classification
     1. Primary
       a. Respiration resumes with stimuli
     2. Secondary
       a. Infant does not respond to stimuli
     3. Treatment for recurring apnea
       a. CPAP 3 to 5 cm H_2O
       b. Aminophylline
       c. Oscillating bed

E. Neonatal oxygen therapy
     1. Maintain PaO_2 50 to 70 mm Hg
     2. PaO_2 > 80 mm Hg associated with retrolental fibroplasia (RLF)
       a. Retinal damage to the neonate resulting in blindness

3. >70% inspired oxygen may result in oxygen toxicity (BPD)

F. Oxygen devices

1. Hood

 a. Keep flow >5 LPM to prevent CO_2 accumulation

 b. May achieve oxygen concentrations up to 95%

 1) High humidity

 2) Aerosol

2. Incubators

 a. Controls temperature, humidity, oxygen concentration

 b. Contain devices to limit oxygen concentrations

 c. For higher achieved oxygen concentration, ports can be occluded

G. CPAP therapy

1. Indications

 a. $PaO_2 < 50$ mm Hg with an $FIO_2 > 0.7$

 b. Secondary apnea

 c. Patent ductus arteriosis

 d. Atelectasis

 e. Hyaline membrane disease

 f. Pulmonary edema

 g. Pulmonary hemorrhage

 h. Hypoxemia resulting from a reduced FRC

2. Methods of administration

 a. Nasal prongs

 b. Face mask; head hood

 c. Endotracheal tube

3. Initial settings
    a. CPAP initially set at 4 to 6 cm H_2O
    b. Use same FIO_2 previous to CPAP therapy
4. Increasing CPAP
    a. When FIO_2 reaches 70%, elevate CPAP incrementally by 2 cm H_2O to achieve a PaO_2 of 50 to 70 mm Hg
    b. Mechanical ventilation indicated if FIO_2 reaches 90% and CPAP is greater than 10 cm H_2O
5. Weaning
    a. Initially decrease FIO_2 slowly and monitor blood gases
    b. Decrease CPAP levels slowly and monitor blood gases
    c. If patient is stable for at least 4 hr on an FIO_2 of 40% and CPAP of 3 cm H_2O,
        1) Discontinue CPAP, place on an FIO_2 of 50%
        2) Obtain blood gases
        3) Chest x-ray

H. Mechanical ventilation
    1. Indications
        a. Respiratory failure with apnea
        b. Secondary apnea while on CPAP
        c. $PaO_2 < 50$ mm Hg; $FIO_2 > 0.9$; CPAP > 10 cm H_2O
    2. Initial settings
        a. IMV mode most common

    b. Inspiratory time of 0.6 to 1.0 sec

    c. Pressure 4 to 6 cm H_2O/lb

    d. Rate initially set at 10 BPM

    e. Control mode rate of 25 BPM

    f. FIO_2

        1) From labor and delivery, 100%

        2) Or same FIO_2 previous to mechanical ventilation

3. Weaning

    a. Increase periods of spontaneous breathing by first reducing the ventilator rate

    b. Reduce FIO_2 as indicated by blood gases

    c. Decrease PEEP by 2 to 3 cm H_2O until a minimum of 2 cm H_2O is reached

    d. Decrease peak pressure in increments of 2 cm H_2O

    e. Monitor blood gases as indicated

        1) Arterial catheter sample

            a) PaO_2 60 to 90 mm Hg

            b) $PaCO_2$ 35 to 45 mm Hg

            c) pH 7.30 to 7.45

        2) Capillary sample

            a) PaO_2 35 to 55 mm Hg

            b) $PaCO_2$ 40 to 50 mm Hg

            c) pH 7.30 to 7.45

    f. Factors to consider while weaning

        1) Spontaneous breathing

        2) Pink color

        3) Absence of x-ray film abnormalities

        4) Absence of chest retractions

III. Neurotrauma

A. Most important factor of treatment in the first 24 to 48 hr is mechanical hyperventilation
   1. Maintaining a $PaCO_2$ of 25 to 30 mm Hg
      a. Decreased $PaCO_2$ results in decreased cerebral blood flow
      b. This results in a decreased intracranial pressure (ICP)
B. During this time, maintain a hyperoxygenated state
   1. Hypoxia causes cerebral vasodilation and increased cerebral blood flow
   2. Hyperventilating to maintain a low $PaCO_2$ causes the oxyhemoglobin curve to shift to the left
      a. This causes an increased affinity of hemoglobin for oxygen
      b. Less available oxygen at the tissue level
C. Use PEEP cautiously
   1. May increase the ICP
   2. Decrease venous return
   3. Decrease cardiac output
D. Complications of neurotrauma
   1. Neurogenic pulmonary edema
      a. Pulmonary edema resulting from cerebral edema
      b. Resulting ARDS possible
E. Treatment of cerebral edema
   1. Use intracranial monitor

    2. Reverse Trendelenburg position
    3. Mannitol to decrease edema by diuresis
F. Stable neurotrauma patient
    1. Continual ventilator dependent
    2. Nursing home
    3. Home care

IV. Nosocomial Infection

A. Hospital-acquired infection
B. Possible causes
    1. Handwashing technique
    2. Contaminated food and water
    3. Aerosol therapy
       a. Bacteria grow well in a humidified environment
C. Frequently cultured bacteria
    1. Pseudomonas
    2. Serratia
    3. Staphylococcus
D. Complications of nosocomial infections
    1. Pleural effusion
    2. Empyema
    3. Cavitating lungs
    4. Pneumonia

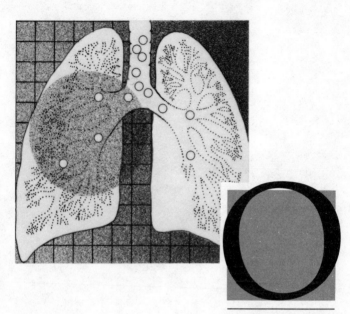

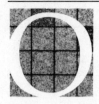

I. Oxygen Analyzers

A. Mass spectrometry
   1. Gases are ionized and separated
   2. Measures true oxygen concentration
B. Pauling (Paramagnetic)
   1. Oxygen alters a magnetic field, which then rotates the dumbbell; the amount of displacement of the dumbbell is proportional to the amount of oxygen present
   2. Uses blue silica to absorb moisture
   3. P_{H_2O} alters readings
   4. N_2 and CO_2 does not affect an accurate reading
   5. Measures the partial pressure of oxygen
C. Thermal conductivity (electrical)
   1. Incorporates a wheatstone bridge
      a. Changes in current are proportional to the cooling of the wire
   2. Pink silica gel provides humidity
   3. Presence of CO_2 gives a false reading
   4. Measures oxygen concentration

D. Electrochemical
  1. Galvanic cell
     a. Life of cell relies on the frequency and duration of use
     b. Contains no batteries (except for alarms)
        1) Response time slower
        2) Electrodes last longer
     c. Reads oxygen partial pressure
     d. Reading affected by
        1) P_{H_2O}
        2) Altitude
        3) Increased pressures
           a) Positive pressure
           b) PEEP
  2. Clark (polarographic)
     a. Batteries polarize the electrodes
        1) Response time faster
        2) Electrodes do not last as long
     b. Reading affected by
        1) P_{H_2O}
        2) Altitude
        3) Increased pressures
     c. Reads oxygen partial pressure
E. Chemical (Scholander)
  1. Measures oxygen by mercury displacement
  2. Measures oxygen concentration

II. *Oxygen Devices*

A. High flow system
  1. Meets all inspiratory demands

2. Venturi devices
   a. Fixed FiO_2 provided along with high gas flows
   b. Can provide 24% to 100% oxygen
3. Advantages
   a. Patient's changing or irregular inspiratory demands does not affect the FiO_2 delivered
   b. Provides controlled temperature and humidity
4. Disadvantages
   a. Back pressure to gas flow increases oxygen concentration
   b. Water in tubing increases oxygen concentration
B. Low flow system
   1. Total gas flow is insufficient to meet all inspiratory demands
   2. Factors affecting FiO_2
      a. Oxygen reservoir
      b. Liter flow per minute
      c. Ventilatory pattern
   3. Nasal cannula or catheter (approximate values)
      a. 1 LPM   24% O_2
      b. 2 LPM   28% O_2
      c. 3 LPM   32% O_2
      d. 4 LPM   36% O_2
      e. 5 LPM   40% O_2
      f. 6 LPM   44% O_2
   4. Oxygen mask (approximate values)
      a. 5 to 6 LPM   40% O_2
      b. 6 to 7 LPM   50% O_2
      c. 7 to 8 LPM   60% O_2

    d. Must maintain a minimal flow of 5 LPM to ensure adequate CO_2 removal

  5. Mask with reservoir (approximate values)

    a. 6 LPM   60% O_2

    b. 7 LPM   70% O_2

    c. 8 LPM   80% O_2

    d. 9 LPM   90% O_2

  6. Nonrebreather

    a. Can deliver up to 100% O_2

    b. Ensure an adequate flow to only partially deflate the bag upon a full inspiration

III. Oxygen Therapy

A. Goals

  1. Alleviate hypoxemia

  2. To decrease the work of breathing

  3. To decrease the work of the heart

B. Physiologic effects

  1. Improved oxygenation

  2. Decreased pulse rate

  3. Improved sensorium

  4. Decreased pulmonary resistance

C. Hazards

  1. Hypoventilation

  2. Absorption atelectasis

  3. Oxygen toxicity

  4. Bronchopulmonary dysplasia (in neonates)

  5. Retrolental fibroplasia (in neonates)

IV. Oxygen Toxicity

A. Complication of long term or high oxygen concentrations

B. Chronic oxygen toxicity
   1. Many months of low oxygen concentration

C. Acute oxygen toxicity
   1. Several days of high oxygen concentration

D. Pathophysiology
   1. Exudative phase; increased capillary permeability
   2. Proliferative phase; development of fibrotic changes
      a. Decreased VC
      b. Decreased surfactant production

E. Clinical signs
   1. Dry cough
   2. Nausea, vomiting
   3. Substernal burning

F. Chest x-ray film reveals scattered atelectatic areas

G. FRC and pulmonary compliance are decreased as in restrictive diseases

V. Oxyhemoglobin (HbO$_2$) Curve

A. Percent of oxygen saturation combined with the hemoglobin sites

B. Conditions that create a shift to the left
   1. Increased pH
   2. Decreased PaCO$_2$

    3. Decreased temperature

    4. Decreased 2,3-DPG (diphosphoglycerate)

    5. Results in an increased affinity of hemoglobin for oxygen

       a. Oxygen not readily released at the tissue level

       b. Increased O_2 content

C. Conditions that create a shift to the right

    1. Decreased pH

    2. Increased $PaCO_2$

    3. Increased temperature

    4. Increased 2,3-DPG (diphosphoglycerate)

    5. Results in a decreased affinity of hemoglobin for oxygen

       a. Oxygen readily released at the tissue level

       b. Decreased O_2 content

D. P_{50}

    1. PO_2 at which 50% of the hemoglobin is combined to oxygen

    2. Normal value 27 mm Hg

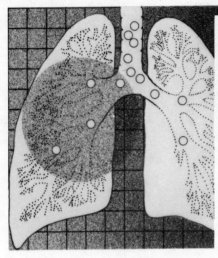

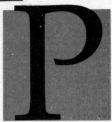

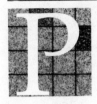

I. Palpation Technique

A. Hands-on-contact with the patient to determine the density of tissue and movement of the thorax

B. Tactile fremitus

   1. Vocal fremitus

      a. Degree of vibrations that are felt when a patient says "99"

      b. Decreased vocal fremitus

         1) Any condition that interferes with sound transmission

            a) Pleural effusion

            b) Pneumothorax

            c) Emphysema

      c. Increased vocal fremitus

         1) Any condition that increases the emission of sound transmission (liquid or solid matters favor sound transmission)

            a) Pneumonia

            b) Atelectasis

      c) Fibrosis

      d) Pulmonary edema

  2. Rhonchal fremitus

    a. Vibrations produced when air passes through an obstruction (sputum, pus, masses)

      1) Bronchitis

      2) Asthma

      3) Foreign body

      4) Tumor

      5) Lesions

  3. Pleural rub fremitus

    a. Grating noise heard when the pleural surfaces are inflamed

    b. A complication of pleural infections or pulmonary infarction

II. Patterns of Respiration

A. Cheyne–Stokes respiration

  1. Increasing–decreasing pattern of ventilation interspersed with periods of apnea

  2. A complication of a lack of cerebral oxygen resulting from impaired cardiovascular performance

B. Biot's breathing

  1. Unpredictable pattern of ventilation with periods of apnea

  2. A complication of severe brain damage with impaired action of the brain's respiratory centers

C. Kussmaul's breathing

1. Severe hyperpnea
2. Presence indicates a metabolic abnormality
   a. Diabetic acidosis
   b. Renal failure

D. Apneusis
   1. Sustained pause at full inspiration
   2. A complication of brain stem infarct with abnormal function of the brain's inspiratory/expiratory centers

E. Sleep apnea
   1. Apnea periods lasting longer than 10 sec and occurring more than 30 times during sleep
   2. Central apnea
      a. Respiratory center failure to initiate inspiration
      b. A complication of encephalitis or brain stem infarct
   3. Obstructive apnea
      a. Apnea occurring from an upper airway obstruction
         1) Tongue
         2) Tonsilar enlargement
         3) Abnormal facial (jaw, nose) defects
      b. Treatment
         1) Nasal CPAP
         2) Surgical intervention

III. Percussion and Postural Drainage

A. Indications
   1. Retained secretions
   2. Post operative patients with prolonged bed rest

B. Goals
   1. Removal of secretions through mobilization
   2. Improved alveolar ventilation

C. Hazards
   1. Undrained empyema
      a. Possible contamination of the opposite lung
   2. Neurosurgical patients
      a. Increased intracranial pressure
   3. Percussing over healing tissue
      a. Pain
      b. Tissue breakdown

D. Body positions
   1. Apical–posterior LUL
      a. Bed: elevated 30°
      b. Patient: one-fourth prone
      c. Percuss: above left scapulae
   2. Posterior RUL
      a. Bed: head of bed (HOB) flat
      b. Patient: one-fourth prone
      c. Percuss: above right scapulae
   3. Apical upper lobes
      a. Bed: elevated 30° to 45°
      b. Patient: semifowlers
      c. Percuss: between clavicles, top of
                     scapulae
   4. Anterior upper lobes
      a. Bed: HOB flat
      b. Patient: supine
      c. Percuss: below clavicles, above nipples

5. Left lingula and RML
   a. Bed: foot of bed (FOB) up 15°
   b. Patient: one-fourth supine
   c. Percuss: below breast tissue
6. Superior basals
   a. Bed: HOB flat
   b. Patient: prone
   c. Percuss: just below scapulae
7. Anterior basals
   a. Bed: FOB up 30°
   b. Patient: supine
   c. Percuss: below nipple, above floating ribs
8. Lateral basals
   a. Bed: FOB up 30°
   b. Patient: sidelying
   c. Percuss: midaxillary line
9. Posterior basals
   a. Bed: FOB up 30°
   b. Patient: prone
   c. Percuss: above floating ribs

E. Technique
   1. Patient placed in proper position
   2. Strike the chest wall on the proper lung segment with cupped hands to produce a clapping sound (traps air between the hand and chest wall; transmits an energy wave that loosens adhered secretions)
   3. After percussing a segment, perform chest vibration
      a. Place the hands on the chest wall and generate a vibratory motion (mobilizes secretions)
      b. Technique performed during exhalation only

IV. Percussion Notes

A. Technique used to determine the type of tone produced when striking the chest

B. Type of notes

1. Resonant
   a. Low-pitched, nonmusical note
   b. Basis for which other notes are compared
   c. Sound emitted from normal chests

2. Hyperresonant
   a. Low-pitched, slightly musical note of moderately long duration
   b. Normally heard in thin-walled adults and children
   c. Presence indicates hyperinflation
      1) Emphysema
      2) Asthma

3. Tympanic
   a. Very high-pitched, musical note of long duration
   b. Normally heard only over the stomach bubble
   c. Abnormal states that produce the tympanic note (air trapped in an enclosed chamber)
      1) Tension pneumothorax
      2) Pulmonary cavity

4. Dull
   a. Moderately high-pitched, nonmusical, muffled note of short duration
   b. Normally heard over the heart, spleen, spine, diaphragm (areas of decreased air content)

    c. Abnormal states that produce the dull note (decreased air content caused by infiltrates, masses, or thickening of membranes)
- 1) Pleural effusion
- 2) Atelectasis
- 3) Pneumonia
- 4) Pulmonary fibrosis
- 5) Pulmonary edema

    d. Can determine the amount of diaphragm movement by percussing at resting expiration *versus* percussing at the end of inspiration

5. Flat (extreme dullness)
- a. High-pitched, thud-type note of short duration
- b. Heard over areas with no air content (shoulders, liver)
- c. Abnormal states that produce a flat note (complete loss of a ventilating section)
  - 1) Pneumonectomy
  - 2) Substantial pleural effusion
  - 3) Substantial atelectasis

V. *Pneumotachographs*

A. Flow-sensing devices used for volume and flow measurements

B. Because they are flow-through rather than flow-accumulation devices, pneumotachographs are better adapted for continuous monitoring

C. Incorporates better frequency responses

D. Accurately measures rapidly changing flow rates
E. Damping is less of a problem
F. Factors affecting read out
    1. Noise
    2. Viscosity of gas
    3. Temperature
    4. Humidity
G. Require frequent calibration
H. Types

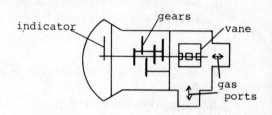

    1. Wright
      a. Vane rotates in presence of gas flow, which
        drives the gear mechanism connected to the
        indicator; registers the amount of volume
        present
      b. Accurate at flows of 3 to 300 LPM
      c. Measurements
        1) V_t
        2) Minute volume
        3) Slow vital capacity
      d. Can use a one-way valve system to prevent
        cross contamination
    2. Fleisch
      a. Within the gas tube, a fixed resistance is
        placed (fiber screen, capillary tubes); the

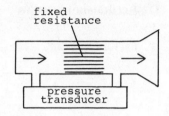

pressure drop across this resistance is measured by a pressure transducer—this measurement is proportional to the flow present

b. Maintains a laminar flow
c. Frequency response depends on the transducer
d. To calibrate, use a known volume of gas injected at varying liter flows

3. Heated element type

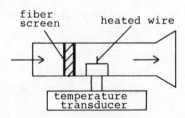

a. Current needed to maintain a preset temperature is proportional to the gas flow present
b. Heated element is usually a platinum wire
c. A fiber screen is placed within the gas flow to protect the heated wire from moisture
d. The signal from the transducers (Fleisch, heated wire element) is converted to volume by integrated circuitry

4. Ultrasonic

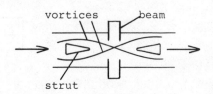

a. Gas flowing over struts placed in tube produce vortices (vortex shedding); these vortices pass through an ultrasonic beam that change the signal to a pulse—the number of pulses produced is proportional to the amount of gas flow
   b. Moisture affects accuracy
I. Pulmonary measurements recorded
   1. Lung volumes (with necessary circuitry)
   2. Pulmonary mechanics
      a. Maximum voluntary ventilation (MVV)
      b. FEV_1
      c. $FEV_1\%$
      d. Flow rate
   3. Tidal volume and minute volume

VI. Positive End Expiratory Pressure (PEEP) Therapy

A. Indications
   1. Refractory hypoxemia
   2. Decreased FRC, compliance
   3. Restrictive diseases

    a. ARDS

    b. Fibrosis

    c. Chest trauma

    d. Pulmonary edema

B. Goals

  1. To correct hypoxemia

  2. Increase FRC

  3. Improve V/Q mismatch

  4. Maintain $PaO_2 > 50$ mm Hg with an $FIO_2 < 0.5$

C. Physiological effects

  1. Increased mean airway pressure

  2. Reduced cardiac output, venous return

  3. Increased lung compliance, FRC

D. Hazards

  1. Barotrauma

  2. Overdistension of alveoli

    a. Increased V_D/V_t (overdistention of normal alveoli)

    b. Increased shunting (overdistention of diseased alveoli)

  3. Increased intracranial pressure

E. Maintenance

  1. Degree of PEEP analyzed continually

  2. Hemodynamic analysis (BP, pulse, CO)

  3. Oxygenation analysis through ABGs

  4. Static compliance

    a. Compliance measurement to assure optimal PEEP

    b. PEEP that produces a decreased compliance is contraindicated

F. Calculating optimal PEEP
1. Best PaO_2
2. Best compliance
3. Best cardiac output
4. Best PvO_2
5. Lowest $A - aDO_2$
6. Lowest Qs/Qt

VII. Pressure Classification: Plasma

A. Plasma hydrostatic pressure
1. Pressure that draws fluid from the capillaries
B. Plasma oncotic pressure
1. Pressure that draws fluid into the capillaries
C. Filtration
1. Occurs when fluid flowing out of the capillaries is greater than fluid flowing into the capillaries
D. Reabsorption
1. Fluid movement into the capillaries is greater than fluid movement out

VIII. Pulmonary Blood Flow

A. Bronchial circulation
1. Supplies the conducting airways down to the terminal bronchioles
2. Originates from the aorta and consists of small systemic arteries

   3. Drains into the pulmonary venous system and bronchial veins

B. Pulmonary circulation

   1. Supplies blood to the respiratory bronchioles, alveolar ducts, alveolar sacs, and alveoli

   2. Originates from the pulmonary artery, then bifurcates at the hilus into a left and right pulmonary artery

   3. Each pulmonary artery subdivide (paralleling the subdivisions of the bronchial tree) and eventually transverse the alveolar capillary bed

   4. The entire cardiac output from the right heart is distributed throughout the pulmonary system

   5. The mean arterial pressure that propels the cardiac output throughout the pulmonary system is approximately 12 mm Hg at rest

   6. Total pulmonary blood volume is approximately 500 ml

   7. Total pulmonary capillary blood volume ranges from 75 ml to 150 ml

   8. Pulmonary blood transit time through the alveolar capillary bed, which is exposed to alveolar air, is approximately 0.75 sec

IX. *Pulmonary Function Interpretation*

A. Ventilation measurements—normals

1. Minute volume	6 LPM
2. Tidal volume	500 ml
3. Respiratory rate	8 to 12 BPM
4. Vital capacity	4.8 L

B. Simple spirometry measurements—normals

1.	FVC	4.8 L
2.	$FEV_1\%$	83%
3.	FEF_{25-75}	4.7 L/sec
4.	$FEF_{200-1200}$	6 L/sec
5.	PEFR	10 L/sec
6.	MVV	170 LPM

C.

		Obstructive	*Restrictive*
1.	TLC	increased	decreased
2.	FRC	increased	decreased
3.	RV	increased	decreased
4.	VC	decreased	decreased
5.	FEV_1	decreased	normal, increased
6.	FEF_{25-75}	decreased	normal
7.	MVV	decreased	normal, decreased
8.	PEFR	normal, decreased	normal, decreased

D. General rule of thumb
 1. Obstructive defects
    a. FRC, TLC, and RV are increased
    b. Flows are decreased
 2. Restrictive defects
    a. FRC, TLC, and VC are decreased
    b. Flows are normal

E. Classification of the severity of obstructive defects

		FEV_1 (L)	*$FEF_{200-1200}$ (L/min)*
1.	Mild	>3	200 to 300
2.	Moderate	2 to 3	100 to 200
3.	Severe	0.5 to 1	20 to 50

F. Classification of the severity of restrictive defects

	VC (% predicted)	TLC (% predicted)
1. Mild	65 to 79	75 to 90
2. Moderate	50 to 65	55 to 75
3. Severe	<30	<50

X. *Pulmonary Function Standards*

A. Flow measuring devices
1. Capable of recording flow within ±0.2 L/sec
2. Range of 0 to 12 L/sec

B. VC
1. Minimum collection device of 7 L
2. Accuracy ±3% or 0.05 L; whichever is greater
3. Flow range of 0 to 12 L/sec
4. Collection time of 60 sec
5. Resistance to flow <1.5 cm H_2O
6. Calibrated with a 3-L super syringe

C. Back extrapolation
1. Less than 10% volume of the FVC
2. Less than 100 ml
3. Whichever is greater

D. Best spirogram
1. Minimum of 3 acceptable tracings
   a. Maximal effort
   b. Without cough
   c. Without glottic closure
   d. No leakage
   e. No false start
   f. No early termination of expiration

       g. End exhalation volume change to be <25 ml
         in 0.5 sec
   2. Must agree within 5% or 100 ml
   3. FVC or FEV_1 may be taken from any one gram
      that has the highest value
   4. May take the largest sum of FVC + FEV_1 from
      any one gram for determination of flows

E. Flow volume loops
   1. $FEF_{50\%}$ may be taken from the largest FVC loop
   2. All other data may be reported from the largest
      sum of FVC + $FEF_{50\%}$

F. DL_{co}
   1. Duplicate tests separated by at least 4 min
   2. Reproducible to within ±5%
   3. Inspired volume >90% of the VC
   4. Breath holding time to remain constant
   5. Breath holding time calculated from mid inspi-
      ration to end of the washout collection

G. FRC
   1. Three tests performed with 10 to 15 min time
      interval between tests
   2. Reproducible to within ±10% or ±200 ml

H. Kymograph
   1. Paper speed of 2 cm/sec
   2. Volume sensitivity 10 ml/L
   3. Flow sensitivity 4 mm/L/sec

XI. Pulmonary Function Tests

A. Nitrogen washout (7 min)
   1. Open circuit FRC measurement

2. Measures N_2 remaining in the lungs after 7 min of breathing 100% O_2
   a. Collection of alveolar gas during the end of the test gives N_2 concentration
3. Normal value <2.5% N_2
4. End of test criteria
   a. After 7 min
   b. N_2 < 1%
   c. Expired volume reached (60 L)
5. Factors affecting washout time
   a. Unstable V_t
   b. Unstable respiratory rate
   c. Hyperventilation
6. Volume correction for tissue N_2 30 to 40 ml/min
7. Duplicate tests should agree within 200 ml
8. Determination of washout curve
   a. Rate
   b. V_t
   c. FRC
   d. V_D
9. Troubleshooting techniques
   a. Minute leaks into the system is the most common error
   b. Malfunction of N_2 analyzer
   c. Leaks at the mouth—sudden rise in end tidal N_2 concentration
   d. Change out of absorbers or mouthpiece can change V_D calculation
10. Comparison to He dilution method
    a. Alveolar N_2 must be assumed
    b. N_2 more soluble in tissues than He

c. Washout test can give a lower value for FRC than He dilution method with obstructive patients; results are comparable if washout time is increased

B. Single breath N_2 elimination (SBN_2)

1. Measures the rise in N_2 concentration from 750 ml to 1250 ml during a full expiration
2. Normal value $< 1.5\%$
3. Test technique
   a. Patient exhales to RV
   b. Then inhales to TLC breathing 100% O_2
   c. Without holding breath, patient slowly and evenly exhales to RV
4. Acceptable curve
   a. Inspired VC and expired VC differ less than 5%
   b. No step change in expired N_2 concentration
5. Four phase tracing
   a. Phase I; deadspace gas
   b. Phase II; mixed deadspace and alveolar gas
   c. Phase III; alveolar gas from both upper and lower lobes
      1) Slope of Phase III
         a) Can indicate abnormal ventilation distribution
         b) SBN_2 measurement (change in $N_{2_{750-1250}}$)
   d. Phase IV; beginning of airway closure in basal regions
      1) Increase in N_2 concentration comes from apical regions
      2) Measurement of the closing volume

6. Measurements calculated
   a. Closing volume (CV)
      1) Volume measured after beginning of Phase IV
      2) Evaluated as a percentage of the VC
      3) Normal CV/VC is <10%
   b. Closing capacity (CC)
      1) RV added to CV
      2) Evaluated as a percentage of the TLC
      3) Normal CC/TLC is 24%
   c. Change in $N_{2750-1250}$
      1) Measures the evenness of ventilation
      2) Normal value < 1.5%
   d. Anatomic V_D
      1) Calculation of Phase I
7. Acceptance of values
   a. Inability to control an expiratory flow of <0.5 L/sec is a major source of error
   b. SBN_2 can underestimate the TLC in obstructive patients
   c. Mean value of three tracings reported

C. He dilution method
   1. Closed-circuit measurement for FRC
   2. Test technique
      a. Patient is connected to the closed circuit at FRC
      b. Patient then breathes a mixture of He until lungs equilibrate
      c. After equilibration, patient does a VC
   3. Correction factor; 100 ml subtracted for He lost to the bloodstream

4. End of test criteria
   a. No change >0.05% over 60 sec

5. Switch error
   a. Patient turned into closed circuit above or below FRC

6. Presence of leaks
   a. Will see a rise in the baseline
   b. No trend toward equilibration
   c. Possible sources
      1) Around mouth
      2) Valve
      3) Perforated eardrum
      4) Connectors
      5) Tubing
      6) Absorbers

7. Troubleshooting
   a. Moisture in He analyzer—erroneous reading
   b. Excessive blower speeds—causes He analyzer artifacts
   c. Exhausted CO_2 absorber
      1) Permits build up of CO_2 in the system
      2) Causes an irregular patient respiratory rate
      3) Causes errors in the He reading
      4) Recalculate VD when changing
   d. Spirometer water level kept constant to provide uniform VD calculations
   e. Leak check
      1) Place weight on bell
      2) Baseline will rise, then stabilize

3) Remove weight—spirometer should return to baseline

D. Body plethysmography

1. Measures the lung volume change within a sealed chamber

2. Incorporates Boyle's law

    a. $P_1V_1 = (P_1 + \text{change in P}) \times (V_1 + \text{change in V})$

3. Measures total gas volume; ventilated or not (TGV)

4. Most accurate measurement of FRC and TLC

5. Patient pants during procedure

    a. Reduces artifacts

    b. Pants with an open glottis and shutter open for airway resistance measurements; open loops

    c. Pants with a closed glottis and shutter closed for FRC and TGV measurements; closed loops

6. Change in volume

    a. Measured by the change in box pressure

    b. Indirectly measured by the change in box volume

    c. Plotted on the horizontal axis

7. Change in pressure

    a. Measured by the change in mouth pressure

    b. Plotted on the vertical axis

    c. Correlates to alveolar pressure

8. Incorporates three transducers

    a. Box pressure

    b. Mouth pressure

    c. Flow at mouth

9. Calibration
   a. Box pressure transducer; use a 30-ml variable-speed oscillating piston pump
   b. Mouth pressure transducer; use a slant-gauge manometer
   c. Flow transducer; use a calibrated rotameter

E. CO diffusing capacity (DL_{co})
   1. Measurement that determines the amount of a diffusion defect
   2. Single breath DL_{co}
      a. Technique
         1) Patient inhales rapidly to TLC from RV 0.3% CO
         2) Patient holds breath for 10 sec
         3) Patient expires rapidly and completely; an alveolar gas sample is collected
      b. Variables
         1) DL_{co} increases with <9 sec breath-holding time
         2) DL_{co} decreases with >10 sec breath-holding time
         3) Patient must inspire to TLC at least 90% of VC
         4) Mean value of three tests reported; must agree within 10%
      c. Normal value 25 ml/min/torr STPD (standard temperature and pressure, dry)
   3. Steady state DL_{co}
      a. Technique
         1) Patient breathes 0.1% CO for several minutes

2) During the last 2 min of the test, exhaled air is collected

b. Sources of error

   1) Irregular respiratory rate
   2) Deadspace of the breathing valve
   3) Increased error possibility in heavy smokers

c. Normal value is slightly less than single-breath value

d. Advantage over single breath is that this method can be used for exercise and stress testing

4. Conditions that create an increased $D_{L_{CO}}$

   a. Increased hemoglobin

      1) The uptake of CO is related to the amount of Hb present

   b. Exercise

      1) Increased blood flow owing to increased pulmonary artery pressure
      2) Results in more blood-filled capillaries

   c. Patient supine during test

      1) Increases perfusion in previously low blood-filled capillaries of the apices

5. Conditions that create a decreased $D_{L_{CO}}$—diffusion defect

   a. Anemia

      1) Deficient red blood cells; reduced Hb

   b. Emphysema

      1) V/Q mismatch with unequal distribution of ventilation

    c. Pulmonary emboli

        1) Reduced alveolar capillary perfusion usually with adequate lung volume

    d. Restrictive diseases

        1) Loss of functioning alveoli through thickening or destruction of the membrane

  6. Bronchitic and asthmatic patients usually have a normal DL_{co}

  7. The DL_{co} can indicate the presence of early interstitial lung disease

F. Water sealed spirometers

  1. Stead-wells

    a. Noncounterbalanced

    b. During inspiration pen moves down

  2. Collins

    a. Counterbalanced

    b. During inspiration pen moves up, bell moves down

  3. Tests performed

    a. Lung volumes

    b. Ventilation studies

    c. Diffusion tests

    d. Pulmonary mechanics

  4. Incorporates a variable speed kymograph

    a. 32 mm/min (1 min between time lines); used with the He dilution test

    b. 160 mm/min (12 sec between time lines); used with the MVV maneuver

    c. 1920 mm/min (1 sec between time lines); used with the FVC maneuver

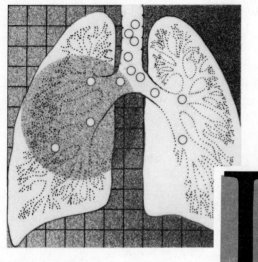

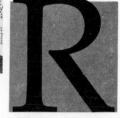

*Regulating and
Recommending
Agencies*

Regulators

*Respiratory
Monitoring*

185

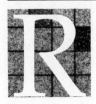

I. Regulating and Recommending Agencies

A. National Fire Protection Agency (NFPA)
1. Installation of piping systems
2. Storage of cylinders
3. Handling of cylinders
4. Grounding of electrical equipment

B. Compressed Gas Association (CGA)
1. Color codes for E cylinders
2. Safety systems
3. Cylinder labels

C. Food and Drug Administration (FDA)
1. Quality of gases
2. Purity of gases

D. Department of Transportation (DOT)
1. Cylinder construction
2. Shipping
3. Hydrostatic testing

II. *Regulators*

A. Reducing valve plus a flowmeter
B. Types
   1. Bourdon regulator
      a. Fixed orifice
      b. Adjustable reducing valve
      c. Resistance placed at the outlet causes an unchanged gauge reading; patient is receiving a reduced flow or none at all
      d. Reads accurately in any position
   2. Reducing valve plus Thorpe flowmeter
      a. Variable orifice
      b. Preset reducing valve
      c. Resistance to outlet
         1) Back pressure compensated; reads accurately
         2) Noncompensated; reads less than patient is actually receiving
      d. Flowmeter requires an upright position

III. *Respiratory Monitoring*

A. Oximetry
   1. Measures the absorption of wavelengths of light emitted by the oxygenated hemoglobin (HbO_2) and the reduced hemoglobin in a tissue sample
   2. Consists of a two-part probe
      a. A light source
         1) Emits a red and an infrared wavelength

b. A photodetector
   1) Converts the light source to an electronic signal
3. HbO_2 is calculated by the change in the red wavelength divided by the change in the infrared wavelength
4. Interfering substances
   a. Carboxyhemoglobin
   b. Increased bilirubin
   c. Cardio-green dye
5. Types of probes
   a. Ear
   b. Finger
   c. Flex (used mainly on neonates)

B. Transcutaneous oxygen ($tcPO_2$)
   1. Principle of operation is the same as the Clark electrode (see Electrodes)
   2. The electrode consists of a circular silver anode that is heated by a coil to produce hyperemia at the skin site
   3. A set of platinum cathodes is placed inside the circular anode
   4. The electrode sensor is covered with a Teflon membrane in which KCl electrolyte solution has been added
   5. A double-membrane is formed by a cellophane membrane positioned on the Teflon membrane, with a drop of KCl electrolyte placed between
   6. PaO_2 is proportional to the flow of current produced between the silver and platinum electrodes

7. A stable gradient usually exists between the $tcPO_2$ and PaO_2 when all factors remain the same (temperature, perfusion, pigmentation)

8. Precautions
   a. Temperature of electrode must be monitored
   b. Electrode must be repositioned every 4 hr to prevent skin burns
   c. Patient must have adequate perfusion to ensure an accurate $tcPO_2$
   d. Electrode should be zeroed and calibrated every 8 hr

C. Transcutaneous CO_2 ($tcPCO_2$)
   1. Measures CO_2 in a tissue sample by infrared absorption or by a modified Severinghaus electrode
   2. Infrared absorption
      a. CO_2 has a specific absorption band (3.5 to 4.7 μ)
      b. The infrared transducer is calibrated for the CO_2 absorption band
      c. Factors affecting the strength of the CO_2 absorption
         1) The concentration of absorbing gases
            a) PH_2O and CO have absorption bands from 2 to 10 μ and may interfere with the CO_2 absorption
            b) The depth of the absorbing layer
            c) Temperature
               (1) Refer to Charles' law
                  (a) When there is an increase in temperature, volume will correspondingly increase; thereby

decreasing the concentration of a gas (CO_2)

 (2) Temperature of the skin site and transducer must be controlled or its value must be known for an accurate tcpCO_2

 d) Total pressure

  (1) Refer to Boyle's law

   (a) Increased total pressure will cause a volume decrease; thereby increasing the concentration of a gas (CO_2)

  (2) Altitude (P$_B$) must be known for an accurate tcpCO_2

d. Contraindications

 1) For an accurate tcpCO_2, the patient must be hemodynamically stable

  a) tcpCO_2 depends on PaCO_2 and blood flow

 2) Debilitated patients

  a) Skin site preparation may irritate tissues beyond healing

 3) Abnormal skin tissue

  a) Dermatitis—increased tcpCO_2

  b) Sclerosis—decreased tcpCO_2

e. Precautions

 1) Patient's temperature taken hourly

 2) Do not cover skin site with blankets, towels, or gauge

  a) Sweating

  b) Leaks at seal

  c) False low tcpCO_2

3) Must maintain a complete seal around the transducer for an accurate $tcpco_2$

D. End tidal CO_2

1. Measures respired CO_2 by infrared absorption (see under [C.] Transcutaneous CO_2 [$tcpco_2$])

2. The infrared sensor must be placed as close to the patient's airway as possible

3. Condensation (giving a false increase end tidal CO_2 measurement) occurs if the sensor is not heated properly

4. The end tidal CO_2 measurement is taken at the peak value at end exhalation

5. End tidal CO_2 may be measured on

   a. Patients who are intubated (oral, nasal, tracheal)

   b. Patients breathing through a mouthpiece

   c. Patients with a tight-fitting face mask

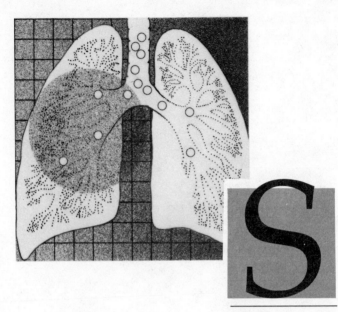

S

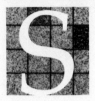

I. Shunt

A. Anatomic shunt
1. Normal shunt that consists within the body
2. Normal value is <5%
3. Causes (veins that bypass the pulmonary system)
   a. Bronchial vein
   b. Pleural vein
   c. Thesbesian vein
B. Shunt effect
1. Perfusion greater than ventilation
2. Usually responds to oxygen therapy
3. Partially ventilated alveoli or increased blood flow contribute to the shunt effect
C. Capillary shunt
1. Nonventilated alveoli in contact with capillary blood flow

    2. Usually does not respond to oxygen therapy
    3. Diseased or collapsed alveoli contribute to a capillary shunt
       a. Decreased ventilation

D. Physiologic shunt
    1. Components
       a. Anatomic shunt
       b. Shunt effect
       c. Capillary shunt

II. *Sputum Analysis*

A. Variables to chart
    1. Volume
    2. Consistency
    3. Color
    4. Presence of purulent material
    5. Presence of blood

B. Characteristic sputum of disease states
    1. Pneumonia
       a. Purulent
       b. Bloody
    2. Bronchiectasis
       a. Purulent
       b. Bloody
       c. Tenacious
       d. Foul smelling
       e. Three-layer type
    3. Pulmonary edema
       a. Bloody
       b. Frothy

4. Asthma
   a. Mucoid
   b. Viscous
   c. Mucopolysaccharide
5. Bronchitis
   a. Mucopurulent
6. Acute infections
   a. Polymorphonuclear cells
C. Collection techniques
   1. Expectoration
   2. Hypertonic induction
   3. Nasotracheal suctioning
   4. Orotracheal suctioning
   5. Transtracheal aspirate
   6. Flexible bronchoscopy
   7. Transthoracic

III. Sterilization Techniques

A. Preparation of equipment
   1. Wash equipment well with an alkaline soap
   2. Rinse well
   3. Let air dry
   4. Package
B. Autoclave
   1. High pressurized steam
   2. Method: denaturation of cells
   3. Uses heat-sensitive indicators to ensure sterilization conditions have been met
   4. Uses biologic indicator to ensure actual sterility of equipment

5. Variables needed to ensure sterilization
   a. Temperature
   b. Time period
   c. Pressure
   d. Strength of pressurized steam
6. Disadvantages
   a. Destruction of rubber or plastic materials
   b. Dulling of sharp-edged instruments

C. Ethylene oxide (ETO)
   1. Method: alkylation of enzyme sites
   2. Uses biologic indicators to ensure actual sterility
   3. Variables needed to ensure sterilization
      a. Time period
      b. Temperature (not >60°C)
      c. Humidity (30% to 50%)
      d. ETO strength
   4. Factors affecting sterilized equipment
      a. Ethylene chlorhydrin: residue remaining after ETO sterilization if equipment had been previously gamma irradiated
      b. Ethylene glycol: sticky residue that forms when equipment is wet prior to ETO
   5. Sufficient aeration time is an important factor prior to equipment use

D. Quaternary compounds
   1. Method: disrupts cell membrane
   2. Effective with gram-positive bacteria only
   3. Solution inactivated by
      a. Dirt
      b. Blood
      c. Protein
   4. Used as a disinfectant only

E. Pasteurization

1. Method of disinfection that applies heat (75°C) for 10 min to equipment immersed in water
2. Does not kill spores, only vegetative bacteria and tuberculosis microbes
3. Equipment must be dried, then packaged upon removal from pasteurizer

F. Glutaraldehyde

1. Cidex
   a. Buffered glutaraldehyde
   b. Disinfection of equipment occurs in 10 min
   c. Sterilization occurs in 10 hr; is sporicidal
2. Sonacide
   a. Unbuffered glutaraldehyde
   b. Sterilization occurs in 1 hr if heated to 60°C
3. All equipment (after immersion) must be completely rinsed to prevent toxic residues
4. Solution effectiveness diminishes after 14 and 28 days, respectively

IV. Suctioning

A. Indications

1. Presence of secretions in ET tube
2. Auscultation of rhonchi
3. Acute appearance of dyspnea
4. Pressure limiting of the ventilator owing to secretions

B. Variable factors

1. Sterile technique maintained at all times
2. Suction time per pass not to exceed 15 sec

    3. Catheter size

        a. Outside diameter (OD) of catheter not to be greater than one-half of the inside diameter (ID) of the tube being suctioned

        b. Equation to determine catheter size: French catheter = tube ID (mm) times 3, then divided by 2

    4. Suction should be done on a prn basis only

    5. Pre and post oxygenation essential with occasional lung hyperinflation

    6. Installation of 5 to 10 ml of normal saline for tenacious secretions

C. Suction pressures

    1. Adult   80 to 120 mm Hg

    2. Child   60 to 80 mm Hg

    3. Infant   40 to 60 mm Hg

D. Hazards

    1. Hypoxemia

    2. Arrhythmias

    3. Hypotension; vagal stimulation of the carina

    4. Decreased heart rate

    5. Lung collapse, atelectasis; resulting from airway occlusion by an oversized catheter

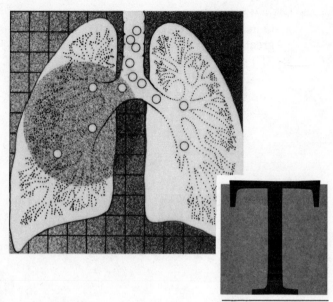

Tracheal Deviation

Tracheostomy

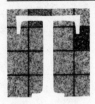

I. Tracheal Deviation

A. Conditions that create tension that pulls the trachea to the abnormal side (affected side)
   1. Atelectasis
   2. Fibrosis
   3. Pneumonectomy
B. Conditions that create tension that pushes the trachea toward the normal size (unaffected side)
   1. Pneumothorax
   2. Pleural effusion
   3. Emphysema

II. Tracheostomy

A. Indications
   1. Bypass an upper airway obstruction
   2. Prolonged mechanical ventilation
   3. Ineffective nasal or oral intubation

B. Complications
   1. Damage to vocal cords
   2. Tracheal edema
   3. Tracheal stenosis
   4. Subcutaneous emphysema
   5. Bleeding at, around, or in the site
      a. Can be life threatening
      b. Exsanguination

C. Tracheostomy care
   1. Inner cannula removed and cleaned every 4 hr for the first 24 hr
      a. Cleansed with hydrogen peroxide
      b. Rinsed with sterile water or normal saline
   2. Dressing changed initially every 2 hr, more often if saturated
      a. Type of drainage noted
      b. Incision inspected
   3. Tracheostomy tube changed every 7 days
      a. Inspect stoma site
      b. Inspect tube itself
      c. Observe for early infection

D. Tracheostomy devices
   1. Trachea button; allows the stoma to be kept patent
   2. Fenestrated trachea tube
      a. Allows the patient to talk and to be evaluated for extubation
      b. Fenestration in outer cannula only
      c. Proper use

         1) Remove inner cannula

         2) Deflate cuff

         3) Cork outer cannula

E. Composition of tracheostomy tubes

   1. Metal

   2. Polyvinyl chloride

   3. Silastic

   4. Nylon

   5. Teflon

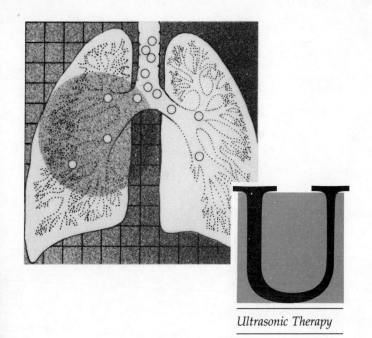

Ultrasonic Therapy

207

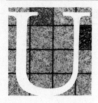

I. Ultrasonic Therapy

A. Indicated for tenacious, retained secretions or for sputum induction

B. An electric current produces sound waves that break water into small particles, the majority of which are 3 to 5 μ

C. Incorporates a piezoelectric disc; changes its shape when a charge is supplied

D. A coupling chamber filled with water holds the ultrasonic transducer

   1. Acts as a transfer unit from the sound waves to the nebulizer chamber

   2. Absorbs the heat produced

E. Nonadjustable frequency (1.35 Mc) of the sound waves determine the particle size

F. Adjustable amplitude of the sound waves determines the output; directly proportional

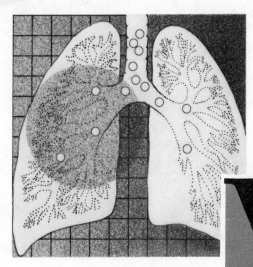

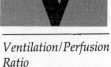

211

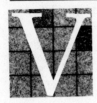

I. Ventilation/Perfusion Ratio

A. Assesses the ventilation to perfusion inequalities of the lung
B. Normal value 0.8
C. Ventilation is greater at the apices; ratio changes to 3.0
D. Perfusion is greater in the basal region; ratio changes to 0.6
E. Increased ratio conditions
   1. Mechanical ventilation (increased ventilation)
   2. Pulmonary embolus (decreased perfusion)
   3. Myocardial infarction (impaired perfusion)
   4. Hemorrhage (decreased perfusion)
F. Decreased ratio conditions
   1. Diseased alveoli (decreased ventilation)
   2. Pneumonia (decreased ventilation)
   3. Atelectasis (decreased ventilation)
   4. Increased blood flow (increased perfusion)
G. V/Q mismatch is the most common cause of hypoxemia

H. Silent unit
   1. Alveoli that is neither perfused nor ventilated

II. Ventilators: Bellows

A. Ma-1
B. Ma-2
C. Ohio 560
D. Monaghan 225/SIMV
E. Siemens Servo

III. Ventilators: Double Circuit

A. Ma-1
B. Ma-2
C. Gill I
D. Ohio 550
E. Monaghan 225/SIMV

IV. Ventilators: Piston

A. Emerson series
B. Searle VVA
C. Bourns LS104-150
D. Engstrom series
E. Gill I

V. Ventilators: Pressure

A. Baby bird
   1. Incorporates a Bird Mark 2
   2. Classification

a.	Power	pneumatic
b.	Modes	IMV/CPAP
c.	Cycling	time
d.	Limit	time
e.	Flow pattern	constant
f.	Pressure limit	10 to 80 cm H_2O
g.	Frequency	4 to 100 BPM
h.	Flow	0 to 30 LPM
i.	I_t	0.4 to 5 sec
j.	E_t	0.4 to 10 sec
k.	PEEP	0 to 20 cm H_2O

3. Alarms
   a. Air failure
   b. Oxygen failure
4. To correct inadvertant PEEP
   a. Decrease flow
   b. Increase the size of the tubing
   c. Adjust expiratory flow gradient

B. BP 200
   1. Classification

a.	Power	pneumatic
b.	Modes	IPPB/IMV/CPAP
c.	Cycling	time
d.	Limit	time
e.	Flow pattern	constant
f.	Pressure limit	10 to 80 cm H_2O
g.	Frequency	1 to 150 BPM
h.	Flow	0 to 20 LPM
i.	I_t	0.2 to 5 sec
j.	I : E	4 : 1 to 1 : 10
k.	PEEP	0 to 20 cm H_2O

    2. Alarms
       a. Oxygen failure
       b. Air failure
       c. Power loss
    3. Has an internal oxygen blender
    4. Adjust I : E ratio when changing rate
    5. Manual breath functions only in the CPAP mode
    6. Minimum expiratory time preset at 0.5 sec

C. Bear Cub
    1. Classification

a. Power	pneumatic
b. Modes	IMV
c. Cycling	time
d. Limit	time
e. Flow pattern	constant
f. Frequency	1 to 150 BPM
g. I_t	0.1 to 3 sec
h. Flow	3 to 30 LPM
i. Pressure limit	0 to 70 cm H_2O
j. PEEP	0 to 20 cm H_2O

    2. Alarms
       a. Oxygen failure
       b. Air failure
       c. Vent inoperative
       d. Power loss
       e. Low pressure
       f. Prolonged pressure
       g. Low PEEP/CPAP

D. Sechrist IV-100
    1. Classification

    a. Power   pneumatic
    b. Modes   IMV/CPAP
    c. Cycling   time
    d. Limit   time
    e. Flow pattern   constant
    f. Frequency   2 to 150 BPM
    g. I_t 0.1 to 3 sec
    h. E_t 0.3 to 30 sec
    i. Flow   0 to 20 LPM
    j. I:E   10:1 to 1:300
    k. Pressure limit   7 to 70 cm H_2O
    l. PEEP   −2 to 15 cm H_2O

2. Alarms
    a. Low Pressure
    b. Air failure
    c. Oxygen failure
    d. Power loss
    e. Failure to cycle
3. PEEP/CPAP system incorporates an OR/NOR fluidic system
4. Manual control button can be used in all modes; sustains inspiratory phase for as long as the button is depressed

VI. Ventilators: Volume

A. Ma-1
   1. Classification
     a. Power   electric
     b. Modes   control, assist, assist/control
     c. Cycling   volume, time, pressure
     d. Limit   volume, pressure

     e. Flow pattern   constant
     f. Frequency   6 to 60 BPM
     g. Tidal volume   100 to 2200 ml
     h. Sensitivity -10 to -0.1 cm H_2O
     i. Pressure limit   10 to 80 cm H_2O
     j. PEEP   0 to 15 cm H_2O
     k. Flow rate   15 to 100 LPM

2. Alarms
    a. Low volume
    b. Oxygen failure
    c. High pressure
    d. Inverse I:E ratio

3. Alarm system for oxygen is a pressure sensor
    a. Red warning light comes on with pressure delivery problems
    b. At 21% O_2, neither red nor green light functions

4. Pressure relief valve preset at 85 cm H_2O

5. Need to adjust sensitivity when increasing or decreasing PEEP

6. Hard to find leaks
    a. Disconnected bacteria filter
    b. Screw loose in humidifier
    c. Torn exhalation mushroom valve

7. If a patient becomes disconnected, the tidal volume bypasses the patient and fills the spirometer on inspiration

B. Ma-2
  1. Classification
    a. Power   electric

b.	Modes	control, assist, assist/control, SIMV, CPAP
c.	Cycling	volume, time, pressure
d.	Limit	volume, pressure
e.	Flow pattern	square
f.	Frequency	0.4 to 60 BPM
g.	Tidal volume	50 to 2200 ml
h.	Sensitivity	-10 to -0.1 cm H_2O
i.	Pressure limit	20 to 120 cm H_2O
j.	PEEP	0 to 45 cm H_2O
k.	Flow rate	15 to 100 LPM

2. Alarms
   a. High and low pressure
   b. Low exhaled volume
   c. Oxygen failure
   d. Inverse ratio
   e. Low PEEP/CPAP
   f. Failure to cycle
3. Incorporates two rate mechanisms
   a. Continuous mandatory ventilation (CMV)
      1) Adjustable rate from 0 or 3 to 60 BPM
   b. SIMV
      1) Adjustable rate from one breath every 3 min to 30 BPM
4. Sensitivity setting is unaffected by the PEEP level
5. If a patient becomes apneic (rate <3 BPM) in an SIMV mode, the ventilator switches to CMV: breaths then given will be the preset CMV rate
   a. Operator must manually reset the ventilator to the SIMV mode again

C. Bennett 7200a

1. Classification

   a. Power — electric
   b. Modes — assist, assist/control, SIMV, CPAP (pressure support optional if ordered)
   c. Cycling — volume, time, pressure
   d. Limit — volume, pressure
   e. Flow pattern — square, descending, sine
   f. Frequency — 0.5 to 70 BPM
   g. Tidal volume — 100 to 2500 ml
   h. Sensitivity — -20 to -0.5 cm H_2O
   i. Pressure limit — 10 to 120 LPM
   j. PEEP — 0 to 45 cm H_2O
   k. Flow rate — 10 to 120 LPM up to 180 LPM demand

2. Alarms

   a. High and low inspiratory pressure
   b. Low exhaled tidal volume
   c. Low PEEP/CPAP
   d. High respiratory rate
   e. Low exhaled minute volume
   f. Low oxygen or air pressure (<35 psig)
   g. Apnea
   h. Vent inoperative

3. Compliance compensation is added to each mandatory breath
4. 100% oxygen available for 2 min (for suctioning)
5. Contains three emergency modes of ventilation

   a. Apnea ventilation

      1) If a patient hasn't initiated a breath

within 60 sec, ventilator continues ventilation from operator's preselected parameters (tidal volume, respiratory rate, peak flow, and oxygen concentration)

b. Disconnect ventilation
   1) Same as for apnea ventilation
c. Backup ventilator
   1) Ventilation continues from factory preset parameters
   2) Occurs when the ventilator detects discrepancies between airway pressure, PEEP, and gas delivery pressure
      a) Disconnected patient circuit
      b) Occluded or kinked tubing

6. Incorporates a safety valve
   a. During ventilator malfunction, safety valve opens
   b. Patient is then able to breathe room air, unassisted by the ventilator

D. Bourns Bear I
   1. Classification
a. Power	electric, pneumatic
b. Modes	control, assist/control, SIMV, CPAP
c. Cycling	volume, time, pressure
d. Limit	volume
e. Flow pattern	constant, decelerating
f. Frequency	0.5 to 60 BPM
g. Tidal volume	100 to 2000 ml
h. Sensitivity	-5 to -1 cm H_2O
i. Pressure limit	0 to 100 cm H_2O

j.	PEEP	0 to 30 cm H_2O
k.	Flow rate	20 to 120 LPM

2. Alarms
    a. Power loss
    b. Low volume
    c. Inverse I : E ratio
    d. Low PEEP/CPAP
    e. High pressure
    f. Low pressure
    g. Vent inoperative
    h. Oxygen failure
3. Pressure relief valve preset at 105 cm H_2O
4. Has an inspiratory pause knob; when activated gives an inspiratory pause from 0 to 2 sec
    a. Cannot use I : E ratio when inspiratory pause is in use
    b. When inspiratory pause is used, vent becomes time cycled
5. Employs vortex shedding pneumotachograph to monitor expired gases

E. Bourns Bear II
    1. Classification

a.	Power	electric, pneumatic
b.	Modes	control, assist/control, SIMV, CPAP
c.	Cycling	volume, time, pressure
d.	Limit	volume
e.	Flow pattern	constant, decelerating
f.	Frequency	0.5 to 60 BPM
g.	Tidal volume	100 to 2000 ml
h.	Pressure limit	0 to 120 cm H_2O

      i. Sensitivity   −5 to −1 cm H_2O

      j. PEEP   0 to 50 cm H_2O

      k. Flow rate   10 to 120 LPM

  2. Alarms

     a. Low volume

     b. Inverse I : E ratio

     c. Low PEEP/CPAP

     d. Oxygen failure

     e. High rate

     f. Low pressure

     g. Vent inoperative

     h. Power loss

  3. Pressure relief valve set at 120 cm H_2O

F. Bourns Bear 5

  1. Classification

     a. Power   electric, pneumatic

     b. Modes   assist, assist/control, SIMV, CPAP pressure support

     c. Cycling   volume, time, pressure

     d. Limit   volume, pressure

     e. Flow pattern   square, accelerating, decelerating, sine

     f. Frequency   0 to 150 BPM

     g. Tidal volume 50 to 2000 ml

     h. Sensitivity   −5 to −0.5 cm H_2O

     i. Pressure limit 0 to 140 cm H_2O

     j. PEEP   0 to 50 cm H_2O

     k. Flow rate   5 to 150 LPM

                   0 to 170 LPM demand flow

2. Alarms
   a. Low exhaled volume
      1) Mandatory
      2) Spontaneous
   b. High and low exhaled minute volume
   c. High and low respiratory rate
   d. High and low peak inspiratory pressure
   e. High and low mean airway pressure
   f. High and low PEEP/CPAP
   g. Inverse I:E ratio
   h. Low oxygen or air pressure (<27 psig)
   i. Vent inoperative
3. Compliance compensation of 0 to 7.5 ml/cm H_2O may be used
4. 100% oxygen available for 3 min (for suctioning)
   a. Automatically resets to preset F_IO_2
5. Integrated graphics page displays flow, pressure, volume on CRT screen
6. Vent inoperative alarm activates if
   a. Temperature control chamber door is open
   b. External flow sensor is improperly installed
   c. Patient circuit is kinked or occluded
7. Cannot increase or decrease PEEP/CPAP during a nebulizer treatment
   a. Ventilator cannot change baseline pressure when a separate gas source is present in the patient circuit
8. Incorporates PEEP maintenance
   a. Flow is increased to maintain desired PEEP level if there is a leak in the patient circuit

    b. Available in all modes except control or time cycle

  9. Bias flow (5 LPM) is present in all modes during the expiratory cycle

    a. Improves oxygen blending during reduced flow rates

    b. Improves detection of delivered and exhaled tidal volumes by the flow sensors

    c. Reduces the patient's inspiratory work of breathing

G. Siemens Servo B

  1. Classification

a.	Power	pneumatic
b.	Modes	assist/control, IMV, CPAP
c.	Cycling	volume, time, pressure
d.	Limit	pressure, volume
e.	Flow pattern	constant, sine wave
f.	Frequency	6 to 60 BPM with assist/control mode
		6 to 60 BPM divided by 2,5,10 on IMV
g.	Minute volume	0.5 to >25 LPM
h.	Pressure limit	0 to 100 cm H_2O
i.	Sensitivity	−20 to +45 cm H_2O
j.	I_t	15%, 20%, 25%, 33%, 50% as determined by rate control
k.	Flow rate	variable

  2. Alarms

    a. High and low minute volume

    b. High pressure

    c. Power loss

    d. 2-min alarm silence

  3. Inspiratory pause not functional during IMV

  4. Peak flow determined by volume setting times inspiratory time percent factor

Inspiratory Time (%)	Factor
50	2
33	3
25	4
20	5
15	6.7

  5. If flow knob not set at infinite setting

    a. Can inhibit exhalation

    b. Can cause inadvertent PEEP

  6. Can give a decelerating flow pattern by limiting working pressure

H. Siemens Servo C

  1. Classification

a. Power	pneumatic
b. Modes	control, assist, assist/control, SIMV CPAP, pressure support
c. Cycling	volume, time, pressure
d. Limit	volume, pressure
e. Flow pattern	constant, accelerating
f. Frequency	5 to 120 BPM
g. Minute volume	0.4 to 40 LPM
h. Pressure limit	0 to 100 cm H_2O

    i. Sensitivity -20 to 0 cm H_2O

    j. I_t 20%, 25%, 33%, 50%

    k. PEEP   0 to 50 cm H_2O

2. Alarms
   a. High pressure
   b. High and low minute volume
   c. Power loss
   d. High and low oxygen concentration
   e. Apnea
3. Peak flow determined by minute volume divided by inspiratory time fraction
4. Volume control knob
   a. To use in control mode, set sensitivity to -20 cm H_2O
   b. To use in a/c mode, set sensitivity at -2 cm H_2O

I. Hamilton Veolar
   1. Classification

a. Power	electric
b. Modes	assist/control, SIMV, CPAP, pressure support
c. Cycling	volume, time, pressure
d. Limit	volume, pressure
e. Flow pattern	square, accelerating, decelerating, sine
f. Frequency	0.5 to 60 BPM
g. Tidal volume	20 to 2000 ml
h. Sensitivity	off or -15 to -1 cm H_2O
i. Pressure limit	0 to 110 cm H_2O
j. PEEP	0 to 50 cm H_2O

    k. Flow rate   0 to 180 LPM

    l. I : E ratio   1 : 4 to 4 : 1

2. Alarms

    a. High pressure

    b. High and low minute volume

    c. High respiratory rate

    d. High and low oxygen concentration

    e. Apnea

    f. Failure to cycle

    g. Low oxygen or air pressure (<29 psig)

    h. Disconnection

3. Compliance compensation is added to each mandatory breath

4. Incorporates two rate mechanisms

    a. Continuous mandatory ventilation (CMV)

        1) Adjustable rate from 5 to 60 BPM

    B. SIMV

        1) Adjustable rate from 0.5 to 30 BPM

5. If a patient becomes apneic, backup ventilation will continue if operator has preset parameters and if the backup ventilation system is turned on

6. Peak flow is indirectly calculated from the tidal volume, inspiratory time, and flow pattern

    a. Peak flow equation

        Peak flow = V_t/I_t (convert ml/sec to LPM)

    b. Square wave

        1) Peak flow calculated times 1

    c. Accelerating or decelerating wave

        1) Peak flow calculated from square wave times 2

    d. Sine wave

       1) Peak flow calculated from square wave times 1.57

Note: For further information about each ventilator (sigh rate, sigh volume, additional modes and options) please refer to specific owner's manual

VII. Ventilators: *Volume* versus *Pressure*

A. Volume ventilators

1. Compensates for changing compliance and airway resistance
2. Does not compensate well for leaks in the system or the patient
3. With obstruction, tidal volumes are maintained with higher pressures being delivered (up to the pressure limit setting)
4. Constant flow generator

B. Pressure ventilators

1. Compensates well for leaks in the system or the patient; useful with uncuffed tubes
2. Does not compensate well for changing compliance or airway resistance
3. With obstruction, pressures decrease
4. The higher the pressures delivered, the less the air entrainment will be; increased FiO_2
5. Peak flows of >80 LPM cannot be delivered with higher pressures
6. Constant pressure generator

VIII. Ventilators: Troubleshooting

A. Leaks in the system
  1. Decreased exhaled volumes
  2. Checks
     a. Tubing
     b. Circuit
     c. Ruptured cuff
     d. Ruptured exhalation valve
     e. Spirometer leaks
     f. Patient disconnection
     g. Ventilator failure
     h. Wet exhaled volume transducer

B. Pressure limit alarming
  1. Kinks in tubing
  2. Increased secretions
  3. Water in tubing
  4. Position of patient

C. High minute volume alarming
  1. Increased respiratory rate
  2. Increased spontaneous tidal volumes
  3. Nebulizer in line; increasing flows

D. Inverse I : E ratio
  1. Check settings
     a. Tidal volume
     b. Peak flow
     c. Rate

E. Patient's breathing not synchronized with the ventilator tidal volume; check sensitivity setting

F. Viscous secretions developing; inadequate humidity

G. Asymmetric chest excursion with tachycardia, anxiety; intubated right main stem

H. Increased dyspnea, diaphoresis, subcutaneous emphysema; pneumothorax possible

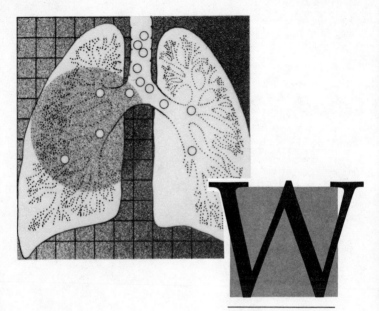

W

Weaning Parameters and Acceptable Values

Weaning Techniques

233

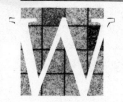

I. Weaning Parameters and Acceptable Values

A. FVC > 10 ml/kg
B. NIF − 20 cm H_2O in 20 sec
C. Spontaneous respiratory rate 12 to 30 BPM
D. Spontaneous minute volume < 10 LPM
E. Spontaneous tidal volume > 250 ml
F. MVV > 2 times the minute volume

II. Weaning Techniques

A. Conventional
　　1. Zero CPAP trials
　　2. Increasing periods of spontaneous breathing
　　3. Alternating with ventilatory support
B. IMV
　　1. Decreasing IMV rates to as low as 1 to 2 BPM
　　2. Increasing the patient's spontaneous breathing
　　　rate
C. T-Piece trials

    1. Time periods of spontaneous breathing with supplemental aerosolized oxygen

D. Factors indicating discontinuance of weaning trials

    1. Pulse increases by 20/min or more
    2. Blood pressure rise or fall of >20 mm Hg systolic
    3. Respiratory rate > 30/min
    4. Tidal volume < 200 ml
    5. Minute volume > 10 LPM
    6. Presence of arrhythmias
    7. $PaCO_2$ > 55 mm Hg
    8. PaO_2 < 60 mm Hg
    9. *pH* < 7.30

E. Factors indicating continuance of weaning trials; initiating extubation

    1. $A - aDO_2$ < 350 mm Hg
    2. Qs/Qt < 20%
    3. VC 10 to 15 ml/kg
    4. NIF − 20 cm H_2O in 20 sec
    5. Spontaneous respiratory rate < 25/min
    6. Spontaneous minute volume < 10 LPM
    7. V_D < 55%
    8. Acceptable ABGs

F. Technique for extubation

    1. Suction below the vocal cords
    2. Suction above the vocal cords
    3. Have the patient deeply inhale
    4. Deflate the cuff while instructing the patient to give a vigorous cough
    5. Quickly remove the tube and place on supplemental O_2

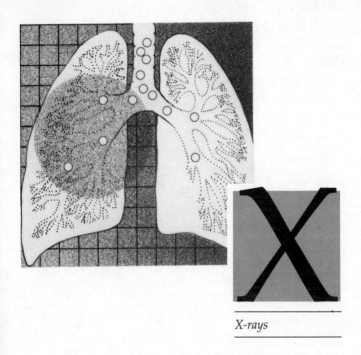

X-rays

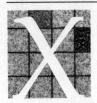

I. X-rays

A. Posterior–anterior view (PA)
   1. Anterior chest closest to film
   2. Used for upright patients
   3. Gives sharpest and smallest cardiac silhouette
   4. Shows clear clavicles
B. Anterior–posterior view (AP)
   1. Posterior chest closest to film
   2. Used for bedridden patients
   3. Gives a larger cardiac silhouette
   4. Shows clear scapulae and vertebrae
C. Radiolucent
   1. Dark areas (aeration) appearing on the x-ray film owing to the ease of passage of radiant energy
D. Radiopaque
   1. White areas (solid masses, fluid) appearing on the x-ray film owing to an obstruction of the passage of radiant energy

E. Characteristic x-ray films of disease states
1. Pneumothorax
   a. Increased radiolucency
   b. Decreased vascular markings
2. Pulmonary edema
   a. Increased radiopacity
   b. Fluffy (butterfly) alveolar pattern
   c. Air bronchogram
3. Pleural effusion
   a. Blunting of costal phrenic angle
   b. Radiopaque outline
4. Pulmonary fibrosis
   a. Fine reticulonodular interstitial infiltrates
   b. Elevated diaphragm
5. ARDS
   a. Diffuse, bilateral alveolar infiltrates
   b. Honeycomb appearance (small cystic spaces)
6. Emphysema
   a. Increased radiolucency (hyperinflation)
   b. Flattening of the diaphragm
7. Lower lobe atelectasis
   a. Increased radiopacity in basal regions
   b. Elevation of the diaphragm
8. IRDS
   a. Ground glass appearance
   b. Air bronchogram
9. Bronchiectasis
   a. Bilateral cavities, some fluid filled

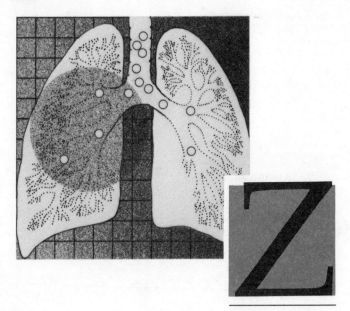

Z-79 Committee

241

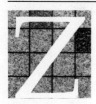

I. Z-79 Committee

A. Developed standards for endotracheal and tracheal tubes and cuffs
B. Specific standards
  1. Bevel of oral tubes at distal end to be 45°
  2. Bevel of nasal tubes at distal end to be 30°; tubes <6 mm in diameter to have a 45° angle
  3. Cuffs
     a. Maximum length from end to end to be <10 mm
     b. Length of tube distal to the end of the cuff to be <13 mm; tubes smaller than 5 mm in diameter, distal end of cuff to be 5 to 6 mm
  4. Packaging
     a. ID printed in lower right front corner
     b. Suggested sterilization method to be printed on cover
     c. Tube marked for oral or nasal use
  5. Only nontoxic materials used

C. Implant testing
  1. Ensures the absence of tissue toxicity
  2. Types
     a. Rabbit muscle implantation
     b. Cell cultures
  3. Nontoxic materials bearing the IT (implant test) marking

Assessment Test

1. An Intensive Care Unit (ICU) patient has episodes of unifocal premature ventricular contractions. You would recommend:
   a. Digitalis
   b. Defibrillation
   c. Quinidine
   d. Lidocaine

2. Causes of a decreased diffusion defect (DL_{CO}) include:
   (I) Anemia
   (II) Pulmonary emboli
   (III) Emphysema
   (IV) Pulmonary fibrosis
   (V) Asthma
   a. I, II
   b. II, III
   c. I, III, V
   d. I, II, III
   e. I, II, III, IV

3. Factors affecting the relative humidity when using a continuous heated aerosol include:

    (I) The length of the wide-bore tubing

    (II) The total flow

    (III) The room temperature

    (IV) The solution level of the reservoir

    (V) The temperature setting of the heater

    a. II only

    b. I, III, V

    c. II, IV, V

    d. II, III, IV, V

    e. All of the above

4. When taking a cuff pressure measurement, you find the cuff pressure to be 20 mm Hg. What system impairment will most likely be present?

    (I) Lymph system

    (II) Arterial system

    (III) Venous system

    a. I only

    b. I, III

    c. I, II

    d. All of the above

5. Normal right ventricle pressure is:

    a. −1 to +7 mm Hg

    b. 15 to 25/0 to 8 mm Hg

    c. 15 to 25/8 to 15 mm Hg

    d. 6 to 12 mm Hg

6. Charles' law states:

    a. With the pressure constant; $V_1/T_1 = V_2/T_2$

    b. With the temperature constant; $V_1P_1 = V_2P_2$

    c. With the volume constant; $P_1/T_1 = P_2/T_2$

    d. With the pressure constant; $V_1T_1 = V_2T_2$

7. An orally intubated patient ha a 7.0-mm endo-tracheal tube. What catheter size would be most appropriate to suction this patient?

    a. 8 French

    b. 10 French

    c. 12 French

    d. 14 French

8. The external intercostals are active during:

    a. Inspiration

    b. Expiration

    c. Neither inspiration nor expiration

    d. Both inspiration and expiration

9. To determine the amount of diaphragm movement during inspiration you would:

    a. Use the palpation technique

    b. Use the percussion technique

    c. Observe visually for movement

    d. Auscultate

10. You notice tall, peaked T-waves with ST depression on the ECG monitor. You would suspect:

    a. Hyperkalemia

    b. Hypokalemia

    c. Hypercalcemia

    d. Hypocalcemia

11. An infant is brought to the emergency room with moderate to severe respiratory distress. Upon examination, you find inspiratory stridor with moderate intercostal retractions. A lateral x-ray

film of the neck shows a normal epiglottis with subglottic narrowing. You should recommend:

  (I) Immediate intubation and ventilation

 (II) Placing the infant in the pediatric ICU and continuous monitoring

(III) Placing the infant on the pediatric floor and continuous monitoring

(IV) Giving racemic epinephrine with cool mist therapy

  a. I, II

  b. I, II, IV

  c. II, IV

  d. III, IV

12. Ethylene chlorhydrin is formed after ethylene oxide (ETO) sterilization by:

  a. Previously gamma irradiated equipment

  b. Equipment that was wet during ETO sterilization

  c. Equipment that was packaged improperly

  d. Equipment that was not cleansed properly prior to ETO sterilization

13. An acceptable tracing for a pulmonary function spirogram includes:

  (I) No false start

 (II) Glottic closure

(III) Maximal effort

(IV) Without cough

 (V) No early termination of expiration

  a. I, III, IV

  b. III, IV, V

c. I, III, IV, V

d. All of the above

14. Diseased or collapsed alveoli will cause what type of shunt?

    a. Anatomic

    b. Shunt effect

    c. Capillary shunt

    d. Physiologic shunt

15. A 0.5% solution contains:

    a. 1 mg : 1 ml

    b. 10 mg : 1 ml

    c. 5 mg : 1 ml

    d. 2 mg : 1 ml

16. Hyperventilating a patient with neurotrauma to maintain a low $PaCO_2$ will cause:

    (I) The oxyhemoglobin curve to shift to the left

    (II) The oxyhemoglobin curve to shift to the right

    (III) An increased affinity of hemoglobin for oxygen

    (IV) A decreased affinity of hemoglobin for oxygen

    a. I, III

    b. II, IV

    c. I, IV

    d. II, III

17. Microorganisms that can cause nosocomial infections include:

    (I) Pseudomonas

    (II) Serratia

(III) Staphylococcus

(IV) Clostridium

a. I only

b. I, III, IV

c. I, II, III

d. All of the above

18. A patient is being ventilated with a Siemens Servo C. He is very agitated and is becoming dyspneic. When you manually bag the patient he seems fine, but when you reconnect him to the ventilator he becomes agitated and dyspneic again. The ventilator settings are SIMV with a rate of 10 BPM; V_t, 900 ml; minute volume, 9 LPM; inspiratory time, 50%; FIO_2, 0.6. You would now:

   (I) Change the ventilator because of malfunction

   (II) Increase the tidal volume

   (III) Increase the FIO_2

   (IV) Double both the minute volume setting and rate control

   (V) Reduce the inspiratory time

   a. I only

   b. II only

   c. III only

   d. III, IV

   e. IV, V

19. What was the cause of the patient's distress in Question 18?

   a. Ventilator malfunction

   b. Patient was deliberately fighting the ventilator

   c. Patient was receiving an inadequate peak flow

d. Patient was hypoxemic and needed an increased FIO_2

20. Double circuit ventilators include:
    (I) Ma-1
    (II) Bear I
    (III) Servo C
    (IV) Monaghan 225/SIMV
    a. I only
    b. I, II
    c. I, II, III
    d. All of the above
    e. I, IV

21. A patient is brought to the emergency room with severe episodes of vomiting. Her blood gases would show:
    a. Metabolic acidosis
    b. Metabolic alkalosis
    c. Respiratory acidosis
    d. Respiratory alkalosis

22. A patient is on 5-cm H_2O mask CPAP. You notice that the CPAP is fluctuating between 2 to 5 cm H_2O. You should:
    a. Get a new apparatus, this one is not functioning properly
    b. Increase the total flow going to the patient
    c. Measure the pressure proximal to the CPAP device

23. Causes of increased deadspace are:
    (I) Pulmonary edema
    (II) Myocardial infarction
    (III) Pneumonia

(IV) Diseased or collapsed alveoli

(V) Pulmonary emboli

a. All of the above

b. I, III, V

c. II, V

d. I, III, IV

24. Variables needed to ensure sterilization during gas sterilization include:

(I) Humidity

(II) Temperature

(III) Strength of steam

(IV) Time period

(V) Pressure

a. I, III, V

b. I, II, IV

c. I, II, III, IV

d. All of the above

25. If the major muscle of ventilation were paralyzed, what percent of movement during inspiration would be lost?

a. 30%

b. 50%

c. 75%

d. 100%

26. The most important factor for Apgar scoring is the:

a. Heart rate

b. Respiratory effort

c. Color

   d. Reflex irritability

   e. Muscle tone

27. Which oxygen analyzers actually measure the partial pressure of oxygen?
    (I) Mass spectrometry
    (II) Pauling
    (III) Thermal conductivity
    (IV) Galvanic cell
    (V) Clark
    a. I only
    b. I, III
    c. II, IV, V
    d. IV, V
    e. All of the above

28. Sodium nitroprusside (Nipride) is indicated for:
    a. Respiratory arrest
    b. Hypocalcemia
    c. Hypotension
    d. Hypertension

29. The central chemoreceptors respond to:
    (I) A decreased PaO_2
    (II) A decreased $PaCO_2$
    (III) An increased $PaCO_2$
    (IV) A decrease in pH of the cerebral spinal fluid
    a. I only
    b. III only
    c. III, IV
    d. II, IV

30. An ICU patient is known to have periods of bradycardia with accompanied hypotension. The drug of choice would be:
    a. Nipride
    b. Atropine
    c. Inderal
    d. Mannitol

31. Find the total flow of 35% oxygen when the flowmeter is running at 5 LPM.
    a. 20 LPM
    b. 25 LPM
    c. 30 LPM
    d. 35 LPM

32. A bedridden 35-year-old woman was noted to be in moderate respiratory distress with hypotension. A PA catheter was implemented. PCWP was 6 mm Hg and PAP was 40/24 mm Hg. The most likely diagnosis would be:
    a. Left heart failure
    b. Pulmonary emboli
    c. Pulmonary edema
    d. Myocardial infarction

33. When measuring exhaled volumes of a ventilator patient, you notice that 50 to 100 ml of the tidal volume is not being returned. Possible causes are:
    (I) Secretions in the airway
    (II) Cascade only one-fourth full
    (III) Nebulizer in line
    (IV) Overinflated cuff

a. I only
b. II only
c. II, III
d. All of the above

34. During the $D_{L_{CO}}$ measurement, you notice that the patient did not hold his breath for a full 10 sec. You would:
    a. Report this test because the $D_{L_{CO}}$ value will not be affected.
    b. Disregard this test because it would show a false increased $D_{L_{CO}}$ value.
    c. Disregard this test because it would show a false decreased $D_{L_{CO}}$ value.

35. When weaning an infant from mechanical ventilation, you would first reduce the:
    a. Pressure setting
    b. PEEP level
    c. Tidal volume
    d. Ventilator rate

36. This flow volume loop is characteristic of:

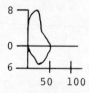

Vertical lines:
Flow (L/sec)
Horizontal lines:
Volume (% FVC)

    a. Obstructive disease
    b. Restrictive disease
    c. Large airway obstruction
    d. Early airway closure

37. What membrane lines each lung?
    a. Visceral pleura
    b. Parietal pleura
    c. Peritoneal pleura
    d. Mediastinal pleura

38. Pushing the diluter in (100% source gas) on a Bird Mark 7 will cause:
    a. Decreased peak flows
    b. Increased peak flows
    c. No change in peak flow

39. An ECG monitor shows a rapid atrial rate with no P waves present. This rhythm is:
    a. Atrial flutter
    b. First degree block
    c. Atrial fibrillation
    d. Ventricular fibrillation

40. Accessory muscles of ventilation include:
    (I) Scalene
    (II) Sternocleidomastoid
    (III) Trapezius
    (IV) Pectoralis
    a. I, II
    b. II only
    c. I, II, III
    d. All of the above

41. Phase II of the SBN_2 test contains:
    a. Alveolar gas from the upper lobes
    b. Mixed deadspace and alveolar gas

    c. Alveolar gas from both upper and lower lobes

    d. Deadspace gas only

42. To correct an inverse I : E ratio you should:

    (I) Increase the peak flow

    (II) Decrease the peak flow

    (III) Increase the rate

    (IV) Decrease the rate

    (V) Decrease the tidal volume

    a. I, III

    b. II, III

    c. I, IV, V

    d. II, IV, V

43. With an F_IO_2 of 40%, the expected PaO_2 would be:

    a. 130 mm Hg

    b. 170 mm Hg

    c. 210 mm Hg

    d. 230 mm Hg

44. Parameters used in calculating optimal PEEP include:

    (I) Lung compliance

    (II) PvO_2

    (III) Qs/Qt

    (IV) $A - aDO_2$

    (V) Airway resistance

    a. I, III

    b. I, III, V

    c. I, II, III

    d. I, II, III, IV

    e. All of the above

45. Causes of excessive bubbling in an underwater sealed drainage system are:

    (I) A leak in the system

    (II) Obstructed tubing

    (III) Presence of a large pneumothorax

    (IV) Increased pressure setting

    a. I, III

    b. IV only

    c. I, III, IV

    d. All of the above

46. A normal pH in a neonate is:

    a. 7.20 to 7.35

    b. 7.30 to 7.45

    c. 7.35 to 7.45

    d. 7.40 to 7.55

47. Organs and vessels contained within the mediastinum include:

    (I) Heart

    (II) Ascending aorta

    (III) Superior vena cavae

    (IV) Thoracic duct

    (V) Inferior vena cavae

    a. I, III, V

    b. I, II, III

    c. I, II, III, IV

    d. All of the above

48. Physiologic effects of mechanical ventilation include:

    (I) Increased mean airway pressure

    (II) Increased dead space

    (III) Decreased cardiac output

    (IV) Decreased venous return

    (V) Decreased urine output

    a. III, IV, V

    b. I, II, III, IV

    c. I, III, IV, V

    d. All of the above

49. The FRC composes what percent of the TLC?

    a. 35%

    b. 40%

    c. 45%

    d. 50%

50. You are giving a mask IPPB treatment with a Bennett PR-2 using 100% source gas. You notice that the oxygen concentration is 20% less than the source gas. Possible causes are:

    (I) Expiratory nebulizer is diluting the source gas

    (II) The diluter is pulled out

    (III) Terminal flow is in use

    a. I only

    b. II only

    c. III only

    d. I, II

    e. All of the above

51. Causes for a greater negative intrapleural pressure in the apical regions of the lung include:

    (I) The apical regions are easier to inflate and ventilate

    (II) The basal regions are easier to inflate and ventilate

    (III) The lungs are gravity dependent

    a. I only
    b. II only
    c. I, III
    d. II, III

52. Complications of inadequate humidity include:

    (I) Atelectasis

    (II) Pneumonia

    (III) Tenacious secretions

    (IV) Bacterial infiltration

    a. I, II, III
    b. III only
    c. II, III
    d. All of the above

53. A patient is given acetylcysteine (Mucomyst) 20% by a hand-held nebulizer for tenacious, retained secretions. During his first treatment he develops a mild case of bronchospasm. You would recommend:

    a. Discontinuance of the Mucomyst treatments
    b. Reducing the Mucomyst strength to 10%
    c. Adding a bronchodilator to the Mucomyst treatment
    d. Using a bronchodilator only

54. Mannitol is indicated for:
    - (I) Pulmonary edema
    - (II) Acute renal failure
    - (III) Respiratory center depression
    - (IV) Increased intracranial pressure
    - a. I only
    - b. II, IV
    - c. I, II
    - d. I, II, IV

55. A patient is admitted to the ICU to rule out possible aspiration. Within the next 24 hr, he develops severe pulmonary edema. You would expect to find:
    - (I) An increased capillary wedge pressure
    - (II) A decreased capillary wedge pressure
    - (III) An increased hydrostatic pressure
    - (IV) A decreased hydrostatic pressure
    - a. I only
    - b. II only
    - c. I, III
    - d. II, IV

56. An arterial–venous gradient is found to be 12 vol%. What hypoxia might be present?
    - a. Anemic
    - b. Circulatory
    - c. Hypoxemic
    - d. Histotoxic

57. Bronchial breath sounds are heard in the left lingular segments of a patient. What conditions might be present?

    (I) Pulmonary edema

    (II) Atelectasis

    (III) Pneumonia

    (IV) Pulmonary infarction

    (V) Pleural effusion

    a. All of the above

    b. I, III, V

    c. II, III

    d. II, III, IV

58. You notice after analyzing a patient's blood gas that this patient has a temperature of 39°C. What would you expect the pH, $PaCO_2$, and PaO_2 to be?

    (I) A higher than actual pH

    (II) A lower than actual pH

    (III) A higher than actual $PaCO_2$ and PaO_2

    (IV) A lower than actual $PaCO_2$ and PaO_2

    a. I, III

    b. II, IV

    c. I, IV

    d. II, III

59. A 4.8-lb neonate needs mechanical ventilation. You would recommend a pressure setting of:

    a. 10 cm H_2O

    b. 15 cm H_2O

    c. 20 cm H_2O

    d. 25 cm H_2O

    e. 30 cm H_2O

60. The volume of air that remains in the lung after a forced expiration is:
    a. RV
    b. ERV
    c. FRC
    d. VC

61. A patient is placed in respiratory isolation. Possible pathogens include:
    (I) Active tuberculosis
    (II) Pertussis
    (III) Staphylococcus
    (IV) Hepatitis
    a. I only
    b. I, III
    c. I, II, III
    d. All of the above

62. Causes of a decreased TLC include:
    (I) Edema
    (II) Atelectasis
    (III) Bronchitis
    (IV) Emphysema
    (V) Pulmonary fibrosis
    a. All of the above
    b. I, II
    c. III, IV
    d. I, II, V

63. The primary sign of hypoxemia is:
    a. Hypertension
    b. Tachycardia

   c. Decreased ventilation

   d. Decreased cardiac output

64. A measurement of the $A - aDO_2$ is 160 mm Hg. You would expect the percent shunt to be:

   a. 4%

   b. 6%

   c. 8%

   d. 10%

   e. 12%

65. A gram-negative rod cultured from an aerosol unit would be:

   a. *Bacillus subtilis*

   b. *Pseudomonas aeruginosa*

   c. *Staphylococcus aureus*

   d. *Streptococcus pneumoniae*

66. Causes of relative anemia are:

   (I) Reduced hemoglobin

   (II) Cyanide poisoning

   (III) Carbon monoxide poisoning

   a. I only

   b. II only

   c. III only

   d. I, III

67. Causes of increased vocal fremitus include:

   (I) Pleural effusion

   (II) Pneumothorax

   (III) Pulmonary edema

   (IV) Atelectasis

   (V) Fibrosis

a. I, II, III
b. III, IV, V
c. I, III, V
d. All of the above

68. Clinical signs of oxygen toxicity include:
    (I) Dry cough
    (II) Nausea
    (III) Vomiting
    (IV) Substernal burning
    a. I, IV
    b. II, III
    c. I, II, III
    d. All of the above

69. When measuring the oxygen concentration of a continuous 40% aerosol unit, you find the oxygen concentration to be 55%. You would:
    a. Decrease the oxygen concentration to 40%
    b. Empty the water in the tubing and reanalyze the oxygen concentration
    c. Increase the flow setting
    d. Change the unit because this one is malfunctioning

70. A patient in ICU has a PAP of 34/18 mm Hg and a PCWP of 18 mm Hg. The most likely diagnosis would be:
    a. Myocardial infarction
    b. Right heart failure
    c. Pulmonary emboli
    d. Hemorrhage

71. The Clark PO_2 electrode contains a:
    a. Mercury/mercurous chloride reference electrode
    b. Silver anode and platinum cathode
    c. Platinum anode and silver cathode
    d. Silver/silver chloride measuring electrode

72. What size endotracheal tube would you recommend for a 6 year old?
    a. 8.0 mm
    b. 7.0 mm
    c. 5.0 mm
    d. 3.5 mm

73. A patient has pulmonary edema. You would expect to find:
    (I) Bronchial breath sounds
    (II) Bronchovesicular breath sounds
    (III) A chest x-ray film with fluffy alveolar infiltrates
    (IV) A chest x-ray film with fine reticulonodular infiltrates
    a. I, III
    b. II, III
    c. II, IV
    d. I, IV

74. The oxygen analyzer that works on the paramagnetic principle is:
    a. Thermal conductivity
    b. Mass spectrometry
    c. Electrochemical
    d. Pauling

75. A pulmonary function test's results show a VC of 3.2 L, an FRC of 2.2 L, and an FEF_{25-75} of 4.9 L/sec. This could indicate the presence of:

    (I) Emphysema

    (II) Bronchitis

    (III) Pulmonary fibrosis

    (IV) Pneumonia

    (V) Asthma

    a. I, II

    b. I, II, V

    c. III, IV

    d. I, III, V

    e. II, III, IV

76. If a ventilator patient has a $PaCO_2$ of 50 mm Hg with a frequency of 15 BPM and a tidal volume of 800 ml, what tidal volume change would you need if you wanted a $PaCO_2$ of 42 mm Hg?

    a. +50 ml

    b. +100 ml

    c. +150 ml

77. In fetal circulation, the ductus arteriosis connects:

    a. The pulmonary artery to the descending aorta

    b. The left ventricle to the aorta

    c. The right atrium to the left atrium

    d. The right atrium to the left ventricle

78. Causes of an increased radiolucent area on a chest x-ray film include:

    (I) Pneumothorax

    (II) Pulmonary edema

    (III) Emphysema

(IV) Atelectasis

(V) Asthma

a. I, III

b. I, III, V

c. I, IV

d. II, III, V

e. All of the above

79. Causes of central apnea include:

(I) Encephalitis

(II) The tongue

(III) Brain stem infarct

(IV) Tonsilar enlargement

a. II only

b. I, III

c. II, IV

d. I, II, III

e. All of the above

80. The type of fungal disease that is endemic to the Southwest is:

a. *Histoplasma capsulatum*

b. *Cryptococcosis neoformans*

c. *Candida albicans*

d. *Coccidioides immitis*

81. Measurements calculated from the SBN$_2$ test include:

(I) Closing volume

(II) Closing capacity

(III) Change in N$_{2750-1250}$

(IV) Anatomic V$_D$

a. I, II
b. III only
c. I, II, III
d. All of the above

82. Equipment that has been immersed in Cidex for over 10 hr has not been sterilized. This could be because:
    a. Cidex does not sterilize equipment
    b. Equipment was not cleaned prior to immersion
    c. The Cidex solution was past the effective date
    d. The Cidex was not heated to 60°C

83. A patient's cardiac output is 7 LPM with a normal $\dot{V}O_2$. What would be the arterial–venous gradient?
    a. 3.64 vol%
    b. 3.57 vol%
    c. 3.49 vol%
    d. 3.37 vol%

84. An unpredictable pattern of ventilation with periods of apnea is:
    a. Cheyne–Stokes respiration
    b. Kussmaul's breathing
    c. Biot's breathing
    d. Apneusis

85. Causes of a dull percussion note include:
    (I) Pleural effusion
    (II) Tension pneumothorax
    (III) Atelectasis

(IV) Pneumonia

(V) Emphysema

a. I, II, III

b. I, III, IV

c. I, III, V

d. All of the above

86. What factors affect the volume output from an aerosol generator?

(I) The size of the particles

(II) The number of particles

(III) The total flow from the unit

(IV) The amount of air entrainment

(V) The patient's minute volume

a. I, III, V

b. II, IV, V

c. I, II, III, IV

d. All of the above

87. The high minute volume alarm has started alarming on a Servo C. The settings are SIMV with a rate of 10 BPM; minute volume, 17.0 LPM; rate, 20 BPM; inspiratory percent, 20. You have just placed a nebulizer in line and checked the breath sounds. The patient and the ventilator seem fine. You would now:

a. Change out the ventilator because of malfunction

b. Change the minute volume and rate setting because of an inadequate peak flow

c. Turn the high volume alarm setting up until you finish the nebulizer treatment

d. Ask the nurse what you should do

88. The air to O_2 ratio of 50% is:
    a. 3:1
    b. 1.7:1
    c. 1:1
    d. 0.6:1

89. Normal value for the 7-min open-circuit washout test is:
    a. <1.0%
    b. <1.5%
    c. <2.0%
    d. <2.5%

90. Possible causes for leaks during the He dilution test are:
    (I) Exhausted CO_2 absorber
    (II) Perforated eardrum
    (III) The valve
    (IV) The tubing
    a. II only
    b. I, III, IV
    c. II, III, IV
    d. All of the above

91. Staining technique used for the mycobacterium species is:
    a. Gram positive
    b. Gram negative
    c. Ziehl–Neelsen
    d. Culture and sensitivity
    e. Transthoracic

92. During palpation of a patient's trachea, you find that the trachea has deviated. Possible causes include:

    (I) Atelectasis

    (II) Pneumothorax

    (III) Emphysema

    (IV) Fibrosis

    (V) Pleural effusion

    a. II only

    b. I, II, IV

    c. I, III, V

    d. I, II

    e. All of the above

93. Particle size of an ultrasonic nebulizer is determined by:

    a. The amplitude setting

    b. The coupling chamber

    c. The frequency

    d. The piezoelectric disk

94. A patient has a respiratory rate of 15 with an I:E ratio of 1:3. The inspiratory time would be:

    a. 0.6 sec

    b. 0.8 sec

    c. 1.0 sec

    d. 1.2 sec

95. Volume ventilators are commonly used on adult patients and not on neonates because:

    a. Volume ventilators compensate well for leaks

    b. Cuffed inflated endotracheal tubes are used in adults and not in neonates

c. Volume ventilators compensate well for changing compliance and airway resistance whereas pressure ventilators do not

d. Volume ventilators maintain lower pressures when obstruction is present

96. The type of percussion note a tension pneumothorax produces is:
    a. Dull
    b. Hyperresonant
    c. Flat
    d. Tympanic

97. Causes of a decreased V/Q ratio include:
    (I) Mechanical ventilation
    (II) Pneumonia
    (III) Diseased alveoli
    (IV) Pulmonary emboli
    (V) Atelectasis
    a. I, IV
    b. II, III, V
    c. II, III
    d. I, III, V
    e. II, III, IV, V

98. You are ventilating a patient with an Ma-1 ventilator. The patient's PaO_2 with an FIO_2 of 0.6 is 67 mm Hg. The physician orders 5-cm H_2O PEEP. After implementing the PEEP, you find the patient is agitated and fighting the ventilator. You would:
    a. Tell the physician that this patient cannot tolerate PEEP therapy

    b. Adjust the peak flow setting

    c. Recommend that the patient be sedated

    d. Adjust the sensitivity setting

99. During a He dilution test, you notice the patient begins to breathe erratically. Possible causes are:

    (I) Moisture in the He analyzer

    (II) Exhausted CO_2 analyzer

    (III) Excessive blower speed

    a. I only

    b. II only

    c. III only

    d. I, II

    e. All of the above

100. You notice that the endotracheal tube has an IT stamped on the package. You would:

    a. Not use this tube because IT means the tube may contain toxic materials

    b. Use this tube because IT means that this tube is nontoxic

    c. Not be concerned because you do not know what IT means

Answers
to
Assessment
Test

Page references in parentheses refer to the text.

1. d (p. 58)	17. c (p. 149)	33. b (p. 92)
2. e (p. 183)	18. e (p. 227)	34. b (p. 182)
3. e (p. 92)	19. c (p. 227)	35. d (p. 147)
4. b (p. 9)	20. e (p. 214)	36. b (p. 109)
5. b (p. 89)	21. b (p. 4)	37. a (p. 110)
6. a (p. 80)	22. b (p. 29)	38. a (p. 102)
7. b (p. 200)	23. c (p. 33)	39. c (p. 60)
8. a (p. 137)	24. b (p. 198)	40. d (p. 138)
9. b (p. 167)	25. c (p. 137)	41. b (p. 178)
10. a (p. 61)	26. a (p. 144)	42. c (p. 132)
11. c (p. 41)	27. c (p. 153)	43. d (p. 67)
12. a (p. 198)	28. d (p. 48)	44. d (p. 172)
13. c (p. 175)	29. c (p. 25)	45. a (p. 26)
14. c (p. 196)	30. b (p. 46)	46. b (p. 147)
15. c (p. 67)	31. c (p. 70)	47. c (p. 133)
16. a (p. 148)	32. b (p. 90)	48. d (p. 131)

49. b (p. 120)
50. c (p. 101)
51. d (p. 104)
52. d (p. 93)
53. c (p. 52)
54. b (p. 48)
55. b (p. 44)
56. b (p. 12)
57. d (p. 20)
58. c (p. 11)
59. d (p. 147)
60. a (p. 121)
61. c (p. 104)
62. d (p. 174)
63. b (p. 93)
64. c (p. 10)
65. b (p. 134)
66. c (p. 94)

67. b (p. 161)
68. d (p. 157)
69. b (p. 155)
70. a (p. 91)
71. b (p. 63)
72. c (p. 65)
73. b (pp. 20, 240)
74. d (p. 153)
75. c (p. 174)
76. c (p. 68)
77. a (p. 143)
78. b (p. 240)
79. b (p. 163)
80. d (p. 137)
81. d (p. 179)
82. c (p. 199)
83. b (p. 66)
84. c (p. 162)

85. b (p. 167)
86. d (p. 7)
87. c (p. 230)
88. b (p. 68)
89. d (p. 177)
90. d (p. 180)
91. c (p. 136)
92. e (p. 203)
93. c (p. 209)
94. c (p. 68)
95. c (p. 229)
96. d (p. 166)
97. b (p. 213)
98. d (p. 218)
99. b (p. 180)
100. b (p. 244)

Bibliography

Alcamo I: Fundamentals of Microbiology. Reading, MA, Addison–Wesley Publishing Co, 1983

Arieff A, DeFronzo R: Fluid, Electrolyte, and Acid-Base Disorders. New York, Churchill Livingstone, 1985

Ayers L, Whipp B, Ziment I: A Guide to the Interpretation of Pulmonary Function Tests, 2nd ed. New York, Pfizer Pharmaceuticals, 1978

Block S: Disinfection, Sterilization and Preservation, 2nd ed. Philadelphia, Lea & Febiger, 1977

Burgess W, Chernick V: Respiratory Therapy in Newborn Infants and Children. New York, Thieme–Stratton, 1982

Burke S: The Composition and Function of Body Fluids, 2nd ed. St. Louis, CV Mosby, 1976

Burton G, Hodgkin J: Respiratory Care: A Guide to Clinical Practice, 2nd ed. Philadelphia, JB Lippincott, 1984

Chaffee E, Lytle I: Basic Physiology and Anatomy, 4th ed. Philadelphia, JB Lippincott, 1980

Cherniack R: Pulmonary Function Testing. Philadelphia, WB Saunders, 1977

Cherniack R, Cherniack L, Naimark A: Respiration in Health and Disease, 2nd ed. Philadelphia, WB Saunders, 1972

Clausen J: Pulmonary Function Testing Guidelines and Controversies: Equipment, Methods, and Normal Values. New York, Academic Press, 1982

Comroe J: The Lung. Chicago, Year Book Medical Publishers, 1962

Davis D: How to Quickly and Accurately Master ECG Interpretation. Philadelphia, JB Lippincott, 1985

Egan D: Fundamentals of Respiratory Therapy, 4th ed. St. Louis, CV Mosby, 1982

Gibson D: Sources of Error in Blood Gas Analysis. Dallas, American Association for Respiratory Therapy, 1978

Hunsinger D et al: Respiratory Technology Procedure and Equipment Manual. Reston, VA, Reston Publishing Co, 1980

Kacmarek R, Dimas S, Mack C: The Essentials of Respiratory Therapy. Chicago, Year Book Medical Publishers, 1979

Kozier B, Erb G: Fundamentals of Nursing: Concepts and Procedures. Reading, MA, Addison–Wesley Publishing Co, 1979

Lehrer S: Understanding Lung Sounds. Philadelphia, WB Saunders, 1984

Lough M, Chatburn R, Schrock W: Handbook of Respiratory Care. Chicago, Year Book Medical Publishers, 1983

Lough M, Doershuk C, Stern R: Pediatric Respiratory Therapy, 2nd ed. Chicago, Year Book Medical Publishers, 1979

Mangiola S, Ritota M: Cardiac Arrhythmias: Practical ECG Interpretation, 2nd ed. Philadelphia, JB Lippincott, 1982

McPherson S: Respiratory Therapy Equipment, 2nd ed. St. Louis, CV Mosby, 1981

Milnor W: Hemodynamics. Baltimore, Williams and Wilkins, 1982

Mitchell R, Petty T: Synopsis of Clinical Pulmonary Disease, 3rd ed. St. Louis, CV Mosby, 1982

Rattenborg C, Via–Reque E: Clinical Use of Mechanical Ventilation. Chicago, Year Book Medical Publishers, 1981

Rau J: Respiratory Therapy Pharmacology. Chicago, Year Book Medical Publishers, 1978

Ruppel G: Manual of Pulmonary Function Testing, 3rd ed. St. Louis, CV Mosby, 1982

Shapiro B, Harrison R, Trout C: Clinical Application of Respiratory Care, 2nd ed. Chicago, Year Book Medical Publishers, 1979

Shapiro B, Harrison R, Walton J: Clinical Application of Blood Gases, 3rd ed. Chicago, Year Book Medical Publishers, 1982

Slonim N, Hamilton L: Respiratory Physiology, 4th ed. St. Louis, CV Mosby, 1981

West J: Respiratory Physiology—The Essentials, 2nd ed. Baltimore, Williams and Wilkins, 1979

Journals

Cooper K, Morrow C: Pulmonary complications associated with head injury. Respiratory Care 29: 263–269, 1984

Sullivan W, Peters G, Enright P: Pneumotachographs: Theory and clinical application. Respiratory Care 29: 736–749, 1984